Lucimar Rodrigues
João G. C. Luz

Repair of mandibular condyle fractures in malnourished rats pr

Lucimar Rodrigues
João G. C. Luz

Repair of mandibular condyle fractures in malnourished rats pr

Assessment and indicators of malnutrition

ScienciaScripts

Cover image: www.ingimage.com

This book is a translation from the original published under ISBN 978-3-330-76305-0.

Publisher:
Sciencia Scripts
is a trademark of
Dodo Books Indian Ocean Ltd. and OmniScriptum S.R.L publishing group

120 High Road, East Finchley, London, N2 9ED, United Kingdom
Str. Armeneasca 28/1, office 1, Chisinau MD-2012, Republic of Moldova, Europe
Managing Directors: Ieva Konstantinova, Victoria Ursu
info@omniscriptum.com

Printed at: see last page
ISBN: 978-620-8-40318-8

DEDICATORY

This boldness has its roots in the past, without which it would have no content, no substance. This boldness, therefore, did not consist in abolishing the past, but in giving it a new meaning, a new relevance.

Neither is ignoring the future out of fear of change, risk and the unknown.

And it's a choice that doesn't lock us into our destiny; on the contrary, it forces us to try the impossible to create happiness in partnership with others, because hope is not lived alone.

And that happiness is closely linked to hope. This way of living our existential project has the property of giving us a unique quality in every moment we live.

Is it too much responsibility?

Yes, but when hope nourishes the days and illuminates the landscape, happiness is a joyful responsibility.

To my dear parents

Aristides (in memory) and Silvina Júlia (in memory)

You have fuelled me with boldness and hope!

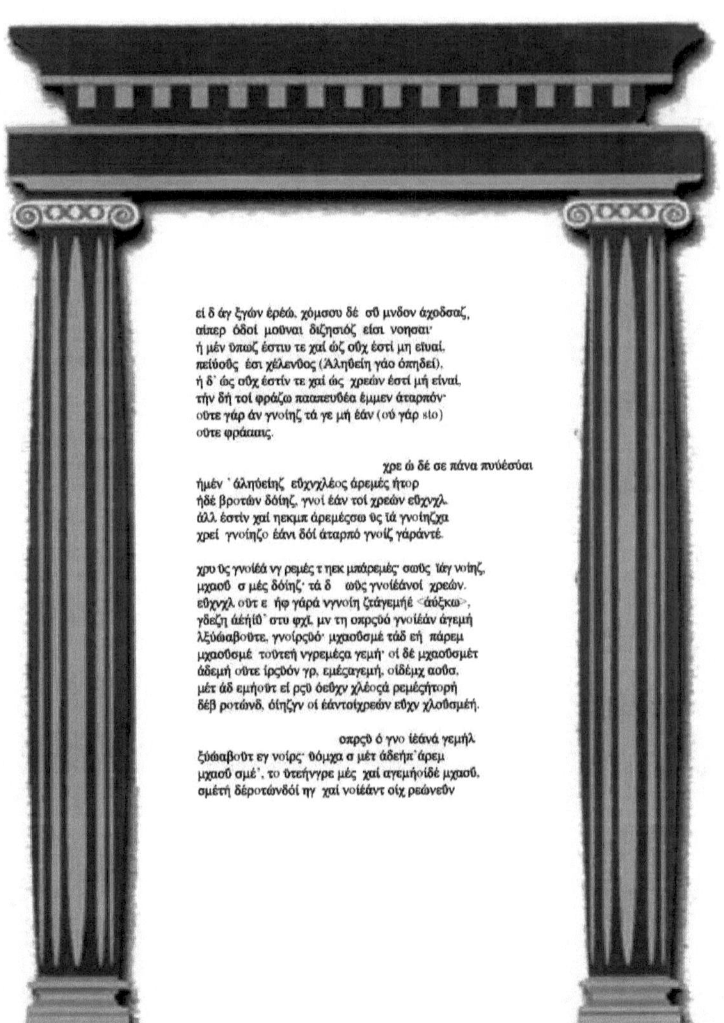
εἰ δ άγ ξγών ἐρέῶ. χόμσου δέ σῦ μνδον άχοδσαζ,
αίπερ όδοί μοῦναι διζησιόζ είσι νοησαι·
ή μέν ὖπωζ έστιυ τε χαί ώζ οῦχ έστί μη εἶυαί.
πείύοῦς έσι χέλενῦος (Άληῦείη γάο όπηδεί),
ή δ᾽ ώς οῦχ έστίν τε χαί ώς χρεών έστί μή είναί,
τήν δή τοί φράζω παaπευῦέα έμμεν άταρπόν·
οῦτε γάρ άν γνοίηζ τά γε μή έάν (ού γάρ sio)
οῦτε φράαιις.
χρε ώ δέ σε πάνα πυύέσύαι
ήμέν ᾽ άληύειηζ εῦχνχλέος άρεμές ήτορ
ήδέ βροτών δόίηζ, γνοί έάν τοί χρεών εῦχνχλ.
άλλ έστίν χαί ηεκμπ άρεμέσσω ῦς ἱά γνοίηζχα
χρεί γνοίηζο έάνι δόί άταρπό γνοίζ γάράντέ.
χρυ ῦς γνοίέά νγ ρεμές τ ηεκ μπάρεμές· σωῦς ἱάγ νοίηζ,
μχαοῦ σ μές δόίηζ· τά δ ωῦς γνοίέάνοί χρεών.
εῦχνχλ οῦτ ε ήφ γάρά νγνοίη ζτάγεμήέ <αύξκω>,
γδεζη άέήίῦ᾽ στυ φχἰ, μν τη σπρςῦά γνοίέάν άγεμή
λξύώαβοῦτε, γνοίρςῦό· μχαοῦσμέ τάδ εή πάρεμ
μχαοῦσμέ τοῦτεή νγρεμέςα γεμή· οί δέ μχαοῦσμέτ
άδεμή οῦτε ίρςῦόν γρ, εμέςαγεμή, οίδέμχ αοῦσ.
μέτ άδ εμήοῦτ εί ρςῦ όεῦχν χλέοςά ρεμέςήτορή
δέβ ροτώνδ, όίηζγν οί έάντοίχρεών εῦχν χλοῦσμέή.
σπρςῦ ό γνο ἱεάνά γεμήλ
ξύώαβοῦτ εγ νοίρς· ῦόμχα σ μέτ άδεήπ᾽άρεμ
μχαοῦ σμέ᾽, το ῦτεήνγρε μές χαί αγεμήοίδέ μχαοῦ.
σμέτή δέροτώνδόί ηγ χαί νοίέάντ οίχ ρεώνεῦν

SPECIAL THANKS

THE TRUTH

(i) The choice

Fr. 2, Proclo in Tim. I,345, 18; Simplicio in Phys. 116,28 (verses 3-8)

"Come along and I'll tell you (and make sure you take my words with you after you've heard them) the only paths of enquiry that are worth thinking about. One, [that] which is and [which] it is impossible for it not to be, is the path of Persuasion (since it is the companion of Truth); the other, [that] which is not and which necessarily does not exist, I declare to you is a totally indiscernible path, since you will not be able to know what it is not - that is not possible - nor express it in words."

PARMENIDES OF ELEIA

Fr. 1, 28-32, Simplicio de caelo 557,25 (taken from 288)

"It behooves you to learn everything, whether it be the unshakeable spirit of the roundabout truth, or the opinions of mortals, in which there is no real trust. But even so, you will learn this too, how what is believed in must be believed in without any doubt, making all things pass through all things."

PARMENIDES OF ELEIA

(ii) The mistake of mortals

Friar 6, Simplicius in Phys. 86, 27-8; 117, 4-13

"What can be said and thought must be; for it is given to be, and not to what is nothing. This I command you to consider, for this is the first path of enquiry, from which I turn you away, therefore, from the path on which mortals who know nothing, two-headed people, wander; for incapacity drives their wandering thoughts into their chests, and they are driven both deaf and blind, dazed, into hordes without discernment, who think that being and not being are and are not the same thing; and that the path they all follow is reversible."

(iii) Evidence of truth

Fr 8, 1-4, Simplicius in Phys. 78, 5; 145, 1

"There is only one path left to speak of: that of what is. On this path there are many indications that what is naive and imperishable exists because it is complete, of one kind, unshakeable and perfect."

PARMENIDES OF ELEIA

TO PROFESSOR DR. JOÃO GUALBERTO DE CERQUEIRA LUZ

The "*choice*" (that of the Truth) was only possible because I was led along paths that were sometimes totally indiscernible.

And in the search for the path "is", it led me to a conclusion as surprising as the result of taking "is not" into consideration. And through it all, without a doubt, what I believe "is".

And on this path, Professor, discerning "is" is an existence in an eternal present, not subject to temporal distinctions of any kind.

If everything that is available to us to think about must exist, and we have to avoid the "is not" path, our only hope as researchers lies in following the "is" *path.* And I will continue to follow your lead.

Thank you.

ACKNOWLEDGEMENTS

To my dear sisters, **Sonia** and **Rosemary**, to my dear brothers **Sineval** and **Itamar**, and to the rest of my family who have been by my side at all times... unconditionally!

To Dr Mário L.S.C de Siqueira, for his collaboration in my daily work and for the privilege of working alongside him.

To Dr Daniela B. Pacheco for her friendship and contribution to finalising this work.

My thanks go to my friends Neuza, Angela and Jussara for their support and help with daily tasks.

Profi. Dr Luciana Correia, a great collaborator and friend, who made the laboratory part of this work possible.

To Prof Dr Antonio Carlos de Campos, for his encouragement and constant support of my work.

To Dr Antonio Salazar Fonseca, for his collaboration and encouragement of my professional development.

To Dr Rogério Bonfante Moraes for his collaboration in the experimental laboratory.

To Juliana M. B. Ghirello for the graphic design and formatting of this work

To Secretary Édison Henrique Vicente, who was always available and took care of the bureaucracy.

To Dr Rita Barradas Barata for her excellent welcome and help in providing information for this research.

To Dr Clarissa Magalhães for the availability of information and teaching material (Food Studies and Research Centre - NEPA - UNICAMP).

To Fundação de Amparo a Pesquisa do Estado de São Paulo - FAPESP for research support (Process No. 2005 / 01891-0).

SUMMARY

This study assessed repair and malnutrition indicators in rats submitted to a unilateral mandibular condyle fracture and protein malnutrition (8% protein with vitamin and mineral supplements). 45 adult male Rattus norvegicus Wistar were used, divided into 3 groups of 15 animals: fractured group, submitted to condylar fracture, with no change in diet (23% protein); fractured malnourished group, submitted to a hypoprotein diet for 30 days and subsequent condylar fracture; malnourished group, with a previous hypoprotein diet for 30 days and maintained until the end of the experiment, without condylar fracture. The amount of feed and water ingested was documented, weight assessed and the coefficient of food efficiency (CEA) obtained. The animals were sacrificed at 24 hours and 7, 15, 30 and 90 days post-operatively. The following blood biochemistry tests were carried out: total proteins, serum albumin, serum calcium, alkaline phosphatase, serum iron and serum creatinine; and a leucogram. Cephalometric measurements were then taken using radiographs of the maxilla and mandible. The histological study included assessment of the fracture site and the temporomandibular joint. The numerical values were subjected to statistical analyses. Feed and water consumption was higher in the de-nourished fractured group in most periods. CEA values were low, especially in the initial periods, and were more significant in the malnourished fractured group. There was little weight gain in the initial periods, except in the malnourished fractured group, which showed significant losses, with weight recovery in the remaining periods, which was significantly lower in this group. Blood biochemistry tests showed a drop, especially in the initial periods, in total protein and albumin values, as well as serum calcium in all periods, which was significant in the malnourished fractured group. The leucogram showed an increase, especially in the initial periods, in leucocytes, lymphocytes and neutrophils, which was more significant in the malnourished fracture group. There was a significant deviation of the mandibular midline from the maxillary midline in the malnourished fractured group, as well as asymmetry of the maxilla and mandible, especially in the final period of the experiment. Histological analysis showed that protein malnutrition led to atrophy of the fibrocartilage of the condyle. Fracture under malnutrition compromised the formation of bone callus, and there was fibrous ankylosis. It was concluded that mandibular condyle fracture in rats with protein malnutrition led to negative changes in total protein, albumin and serum calcium values, leukocytosis, as well as compromised bone callus formation and induced fibrocartilage atrophy and fibrous ankylosis.

Keywords: Mandibular condyle - Protein-energy malnutrition - Repair. Mandibular Fractures - Bone Repair

SUMMARY

CHAPTER 1

INTRODUCTION

Among the fractures of the maxillomandibular complex, fractures of the mandibular condyle are one of the most common. These can be related to injuries to the temporomandibular joint (TMJ) and masticatory muscles. However, the great capacity of the TMJ to repair itself has been demonstrated in experimental models in rats in the face of trauma. This adaptive capacity may be conditioned to environmental alterations, mainly dietary components, and at the same time, pathological processes in its tissues may also determine significant endogenous systemic alterations, since it involves one of the most demanded joints in the body. However, in experimental models of this fracture in rats, a substantial loss of body weight has been observed in the animals. This weight loss has been attributed to difficulty chewing. The possibility that weight loss may be related to a state of malnutrition and that this state may interfere with the bone repair process, slowing it down, should be considered and investigated.

According to the World Health Organisation, malnutrition is a condition of protein-calorie deficiency that includes severe forms of the disease, such as marasmus (insufficient calorie supply) and Kwashiorkor (severe protein deprivation), as well as phases and moderate forms (WHO, 1962). It is estimated that malnutrition affects between half and two thirds of the world's population (YUNES, 1976). It has been reported that for every one child who dies from energy-protein malnutrition, another six survive in hunger and disease (UNICEF, 1994). Protein-energy malnutrition affects children from poor communities to elderly patients, potentiating infectious processes and increasing the number of deaths (CHANDRA, 1999).

Fracture healing is a specialised response in which the regeneration of bone tissue restores integrity to the skeleton. Although the majority of fractures heal without major difficulties, there are certain conditions under which reducing the time taken for the healing process, as well as improving its quality, would be of great benefit in ensuring the rapid restoration of function and improving the physical and mental well-being of patients. In addition, nutritional status should be considered as an influential factor in fracture healing, as bone and tissue repair depend on it. Protein malnutrition, which is widespread in Brazil, can negatively affect fracture healing (GUARNIERO et al., 1992).

It is therefore important to experimentally study the repair process of mandibular condyle fractures under conditions of protein malnutrition, in parallel with malnutrition indicators.

CHAPTER 2

LITERATURE REVIEW

2.1 Occurrence of mandibular condyle fractures and their effects

Koski (1968) reviewed the role of craniofacial growth centres and stated that, based on current knowledge, most of them cannot be qualified as such. In principle, it has been described that the cartilage of the mandibular condyle is responsible for the anteroposterior growth of the mandible, constituting an important growth centre, as well as being highly responsive to mechanical stimuli. However, he stated that the condylar cartilage is not the most important centre of mandibular growth, which has been demonstrated in experimental studies using condylectomies. Mandibular growth occurs through periosteal and endosteal apposition, as well as resorption and remodelling, and is made up of relatively independent parts, dependent on different factors. Therefore, in the absence of a mandibular condyle, even though deformities occur in the mandible, especially in the posterior portion of the ramus, muscle action or another type of force will be responsible for compensating growth.

In their series of mandibular fractures, Larsen and Nielsen (1976) found that the most frequent site was the region of the condylar process.

Enlow et al. (1977) emphasised the role of occlusal intercuspation in controlling craniofacial morphogenesis. Thus, when an extraoral traction is applied only to the maxilla, displacing it in a posterior direction, a similar displacement occurs in the mandible. The same phenomenon is seen when the force is applied to the mandible and the maxilla is displaced together, probably through intercuspation. Similarly, when the condyle fails to disarticulate, as occurs in fibrous ankylosis, all facial growth becomes distorted, probably due to the same phenomenon.

Lindahl (1977) reported on the characteristics of mandibular condyle fractures through his casuistry. He described a medial angulation of the fragment, with a tendency for the fracture line to ride in adult individuals.

Proffit, Vig and Turvey (1980) reported, based on their clinical experience, that a history of condylar fracture may be related to 5 to 10 per cent of cases of mandibular underdevelopment and asymmetries. This is often due to the absence of signs immediately after the trauma and a lack of diagnosis during the growth phase. They stated that condylar fractures may be more frequent than believed.

Pinkert (1982) histologically analysed the behaviour of the articular disc in condylar fractures with deviation in cadavers. He found that the disc moves along with the condyle and remains associated with it.

Winstanley (1984) stated that in condylar fractures the fragment moves medially due to movement of the ascending ramus.

Lindqvist et al. (1986) reported on facial fractures resulting from bicycle accidents, where condylar fractures accounted for 67% of mandibular fractures. Unilateral fractures were the most frequent. They stated that if condylar fractures generally result from indirect trauma, falls with trauma to the mental region are the most likely cause and that the most frequent victims are children, this could represent the potential occurrence of growth disorders.

Amaratunga (1987) reported on condylar fractures. He found that these accounted for 40.0% of mandibular fractures and 71.7% occurred in isolation. Unilateral fractures were more common.

Belli et al. (1987) reported on their series of condylar fractures. These were more frequent in the 15 to 20 year age group and most were isolated and unilateral.

Cormack (1987) described the events that follow a fracture. Initially, bleeding occurs, with collagen formation. With the interruption of the haversian systems, necrosis occurs near the stumps. Repair begins with the proliferation, from the periosteum, of cartilaginous and bone tissue next to the fracture trace. These tissues then fuse, uniting the fragments. The cartilage is replaced by bone tissue and the necrotic bone is resorbed. Finally, the peripheral cancellous bone is transformed into compact bone.

Goss and Bosanquet (1990) reported on aspects of the TMJ after acute trauma, using arthroscopy in patients with mandibular fractures. They found a high frequency of lesions, especially haemarthrosis with laceration of the articular disc and articular surfaces. The most intense injuries occurred when there was no condylar fracture.

Ayoub and Mostafa (1992) assessed six patients with condylar abnormalities. They found that the mandible showed posterior rotation and deficient length in the body and ascending ramus. With regard to condylar fractures, they stated that the altered condylar position affects the mandibular growth pattern, resulting in asymmetry.

Silvennoinen et al. (1992) described that condylar fractures accounted for 52.4% of mandibular fractures. Regarding the location of condylar fractures, 71.5% were unilateral, 19% with displacement and 8% without displacement.

Successful treatment of condylar process fractures depends on the biological character and adaptive capacity of the masticatory system. This will differ in each patient and systemic alterations may lead to an unfavourable outcome. Therefore, predicting the prognosis and carrying out the appropriate treatment will result in benefits for the patient. Bilateral condylar fractures require more extensive adaptations to the masticatory system, but have more favourable results compared to unilateral condylar fractures. After treatment of the fracture, adaptations of the muscles, skeleton and dentition will occur, and may show visible changes such as a decrease in the mandibular plane. Surgical treatment of condylar fractures can favour functional outcomes. However, the risks are not only surgical, but biological, as the disruption of the blood supply to the condyle can lead to resorption/remodelling (ELLIS; THROCKMORTON, 2005).

Manganello-Souza and Luz (2006) stated that condylar fractures are more common than in other regions of the mandible. The most common form is medial displacement of the proximal fragment (condyle) by the lateral pterygoid muscle.

Andersson, Hallmer and Eriksson (2007) recorded all mandibular fractures from 1972 to 1976 in the city of Malmo, Sweden. In 2005, they investigated all patients treated without surgery for unilateral mandibular condyle fractures without displacement and with minor displacement. During this period, out of a total of 49 cases, 23 were assessed subsequently. The follow-up checked the occurrence of symptoms such as pain, headache, masticatory function and the occurrence of joint noises. The results showed that 87 per cent of the patients had no pain, 83 per cent had no problems with masticatory function and 91 per cent had no problems with daily activities. They had neck and shoulder symptoms (39 per cent) and back pain (30 per cent). After 31 years, the non-surgical treatment of unilateral condylar fractures seems to be favourable in terms of function, occurrence of pain and difficulty in daily activities.

2.2 Experimental models

Das, Meyer and Sicher (1965) carried out a radiographic study of the mandible of young rats to analyse the effects of bilateral condylectomy. They used the lateral view of the hemi-mandibles for measurements. They found that there was a change in growth with excessive bone apposition in areas of muscle insertion, especially in the mandibular angle due to muscle hypertrophy. They considered adapted growth of the mandible with normal size but altered shapes.

Gianelly and Moorrees (1965) carried out an experimental study to assess the contribution of the condyle to the growth of the mandible in young rats submitted to bilateral condylectomy; one group as an operated control and one control group. Radiographs were taken using a lateral view of the skull and the anteroposterior length of the mandible was measured. The result was a reduction in the length of the mandible in the condylectomised group when compared to the control group, and the occlusal relationship between the maxilla and mandible was not altered.

Boyne (1967) experimentally performed condylar fractures in monkeys, using osteotomies in the neck region. After a period of eight to 16 weeks, he histologically verified the abundant formation of bone callus at the fracture site. The condyle showed intense activity, with areas of bone remodelling and cartilage proliferation.

Models of facial fractures using animals, mainly rats, have been used since the 70s. These studies sought to clarify the process of bone repair in facial bones under various experimental conditions, such as a fracture followed by detachment of the lateral pterygoid muscle (SPRINZ, 1970).

Gilhuus-Moe (1971) experimentally performed a unilateral condylar fracture with deviation in guinea pigs. Histopathological and auto-radiographic studies showed an increase in the activity of the intermediate (proliferative) layer of the condyle on both sides. He concluded that this phenomenon is due to the intense adaptability of the mandibular condyle.

Craft et al. (1974) histologically studied the repair process of experimental mandibular and zygomatic arch fractures in rabbits. They observed that after one week, osteoid tissue was present from the periosteum; at two weeks, chondroid tissue in the fracture trace and osteoid in the periphery; at three weeks, the presence of callus basically of trabecular bone; at four weeks, re-modelling in cortical bone.

Banks and Mackenzie (1975) performed subcondylar osteotomies without deviation in adult monkeys. After three to 12 months, they observed medial displacement of the condyle. Histologically, they observed signs of remodelling near the insertion of the lateral pterygoid muscle in the initial periods. The authors believe that this muscle remodels its insertion, returning to its normal alignment.

Ahmed et al. (1978) compared the effects of open or closed reduction in the treatment of condylar fractures during the growth period in dogs. After periods of six to 18 months, they observed a significant difference between the operated and control sides in the height of the ascending ramus of the mandible. Histological analysis of the articular surface revealed a progressive decrease in the thickness of the fibrocartilage. The results showed no significant difference between the treatment methods, although the changes were greater in the group with open reduction.

Markey, Potter and Moffett (1980) performed condylar fractures on young monkeys with prolonged maxillo-mandibular block. Using metal markers, they verified the occurrence of asymmetry. There was deviation and limited mouth opening, which recovered in a few months. They concluded that other factors complicating pre-existing trauma could lead to TMJ ankylosis.

Shimahara, Ono and Nakano (1985) experimentally fractured the unilateral condyle without deviation in rats and compared the results obtained without an intermaxillary block and with a block for one week and five weeks. The group fractured with a block showed poor weight gain for 5 weeks. Histological examination showed an intense initial inflammatory response and, after five weeks, the fractured group without blockade showed repair by cartilaginous proliferation, but the fractured group with blockade showed intramembranous ossification in one week and in the fifth week showed medial displacement of the fragment together with intramembranous ossification.

Granstrom and Nilsson (1987) histologically assessed the repair process of experimental mandibular fractures in rats. They found that initially the fracture area was filled with granulation tissue, with resorption of the bone stumps; at four days there was bone proliferation from the periosteum, and at six days from the compact bone; at eight days cartilaginous tissue was observed in the fracture trace; at ten days bone callus had formed around the fracture line; at 14 days there were bone trabeculae in the fracture line; at 16 days there was resorption of the newly formed cartilage; at 24 days the fracture site was completely filled with bone trabeculae and there was remodelling of the bone callus.

Shimahara et al. (1987) experimentally performed a unilateral condylar fracture with deviation in rats, a position maintained by osteosynthesis for one month. Macroscopically, there was midline deviation in some of the animals and the condyle showed deviation and a change in shape for up to four months, tending to return to its normal position at eight months. The animals gained weight. Histologically, they observed repair by cartilaginous and bone proliferation at two months, with remodelling in the neck region at eight months.

Mabuchi (1988) evaluated the effects of unilateral mandibular fractures on the condyles of newborn rats. Repair of the fracture began with the deposition of granulation tissue at three days, followed by bone neoformation beginning at nine days and more intense at 15 and 21 days. There was a decrease in the cellularity and thickness of all the layers that make up the articular fibrocartilage, on both sides.

The mandibular condyle is a synovial joint that is one of the growth centres of the face. For this reason, it has a high capacity for functional adaptation and is one of the models of choice for studying growth and cartilage and bone remodelling. Livne and Silbermann (1990) describe that, during the neonatal period, the condyle undergoes endochondral ossification generating elongation of the mandibular ramus; subsequently, a fibrous connective tissue appears at the site, as the cartilage becomes hypotrophic; at this stage, compact bone tissue is already seen around the cartilaginous tissue. Two main cellular compartments are described for the condyle: the chondroprogenitor zone, formed by mesenchymal-like cells (with elongated cytoplasmic processes and pronounced cell-cell contact) not normally seen in other synovial joints; and a cartilaginous zone, containing cartilaginous cells at different stages of maturation. The authors conclude that the mouse condyle is an excellent model for studying cartilage growth and remodelling, as well as the effects of ageing on this tissue.

Luz et al. (1991) histologically assessed the effects of indirect trauma on the TMJ in a model using rats. They used adult rats subjected to indirect trauma to the TMJ on the right side, with the left side as a control. They found that despite the trauma, the animals had increased weight and none of them had limited mouth opening. The data showed that the impact could produce a fracture in the mandibular fossa and lesions on the articular surface of the condyle and the articular disc. Initially, there was an acute inflammatory process. Subsequently, they observed signs of a proliferative response from the articular surfaces. After one month there were signs of bone remodelling in the mandibular ramus and after three months, joint structures with normal characteristics and signs of remodelling were observed.

Yasuoka and Oka (1991) carried out a histomorphometric study of the repair process of an experimental condyle fracture without deviation in rats during the growth phase. Histologically, they verified the formation of bone callus, with complete union with trabecular bone observed after eight weeks. Morphometry showed a significant increase in bone volume in the initial phases, a significant increase in the areas of osteoids and osteoblasts at the beginning and an increase in the areas of resorption at the end of the experiment. They concluded that bone remodelling plays an important role in the repair of condylar fractures in the growth phase.

Monje et al. (1993) experimentally performed subcondylar osteotomy on young and adult rats. After 20 to 60 days, they radiographically observed antero-inferior displacement of the condyle in the young animals, with slight anterior displacement in the adult animals. Histologically, they observed signs of joint remodelling in both groups, with fibrosis and bone resorption occurring in the adult animals. There were no histological changes in the control-operated animals.

Suuronen et al. (1994) evaluated the effects of osteotomy and screw osteosynthesis on the mandibular condyle experimentally in sheep. Radiographically, they found bone destruction, osteophytes and flattening of the condyle. Histologically, they observed thickening of the condylar cartilage, with imprecise boundaries between its layers.

In an experimental study, Yamamoto, Novelli and Luz (1997) performed a unilateral upper incisor extraction in young rats and analysed its effects on facial growth. For cephalometric assessment, axial and rostro-caudal views were taken of the fixed skull, as well as axial and lateral views of the hemi-mandibles after dissection. The measurements were made using a computer system. In the axial view, a line was drawn joining the tympanic bullae and the midline of the maxilla and mandible, while in the rostro-caudal view, points such as the zygomatic arch and antegonal notch were used. In the axial view after dissection, measurements were made between the tympanic bulla, mesial root of the first molar, in- fra-orbital foramen and incisal point. In the lateral view of the hemi-jaws, the incisor insertion, condylar process, angular process, distal face of the third molar and antegonal notch were used. Facial asymmetry was observed only in the anterior region of the maxilla, with a deviation towards the operated side.

Goulart et al. (1998) in an experimental study with young rats, analysed the effects of a unilateral fracture with medial deviation of the zygomatic arch during the growth period. Axial and rostro-caudal views of the fixed skull were taken. In the axial view, the depth of the infratemporal fossa was measured using the distance between the medial cortex of the zygomatic arch and the lateral cortex of the mandible and the distance between the median plane and the lower incisors using perpendiculars of the midpoints between the tympanic bullae and the lower incisors. In the rostro-caudal view, the distance between the zygomatic arch and the mandible was measured between the point of greatest radiopacity of the zygomatic arch and the lateral cortex of the ramus of the mandible. They observed a significant difference in the depth of the in- fratemporal fossa, and no alterations were found in the other measurements.

Teixeira et al. (1998) assessed the process of condylar repair after unilateral fracture followed by rotational deviation in adult rats. The authors found that in the first week after the fracture, the animals showed some weight loss, which was gradually recovered over the course of the experiment, which ended 3 months after the fracture. In the morphological analysis of the TMJ, the authors found serofibrinous exudate in the joint space 24 hours after the fracture and acute inflammation in the joint capsule and surrounding muscle fibres; bone and cartilage proliferation was seen on the external surface of the fracture after one week, as well as signs of osteoclastic resorption around the fracture line and devitalised bone in this region; at two weeks there was bone callus formation on the fracture line and granulation tissue on the articular surface; at one month of the experiment, the authors found neoformed bone, a reduction in cartilage and discrete remnants of necrotic bone tissue; in the articular space, the presence of connective tissue was recorded; finally, at 3 months the condylar process showed normal characteristics, with basophilic lines of apposition in the subcondylar region indicative of remodelling.

In an experimental study, Rocha et al. (1999) performed a unilateral fracture of the zygomatic arch in young rats and analysed the effects on facial growth. Axial views of the dry skull and lateral views of the hemi-mandibles were taken. In the axial view, they used points such as the lateral cortex of the skull, the medial cortex of the zygomatic arch, the tympanic bulla, the mesial root of the first molar, the infraorbital foramen and the incisal point. In the lateral view of the hemi-jaws, they used the condylar process, angular process, distal face of the third molar, antegonial notch and incisor insertion. They observed a smaller difference for the height of the body and ramus of the mandible, with no difference for the other measurements.

In an experimental study, Luz and Araújo (2001) evaluated unilateral subcondylar fractures followed by rotation in young rats. Cephalometric measurements were taken to assess the angle of deviation of the mandibular midline. They found facial asymmetry with more pronounced mandibular deviation in the experimental group. The authors observed that, one week after the fracture, the fractured animals showed a significant reduction in body weight, which increased in a fortnight and decreased significantly again one month after the fracture. In the end, body weight recovered, but it was lower than that of the animals without condylar fractures. Histological data initially showed neutrophilic and serofibrinous exudation near the fracture trace. One week later, areas of proliferation of cartilaginous and bone tissue were observed near the fracture site. Two weeks later, exuberant bone callus formation was seen. One month later, the condylar process showed normal characteristics and was centred in the mandibular fossa, the same finding observed at three months. The authors point out that the condylar fracture had some influence on the masticatory capacity of the animals, which were still in the period of condylar growth. The authors concluded that condylar repair in young rats occurs more quickly and effectively than in adult rats.

Rodrigues and Luz (2001) carried out an experimental study to assess the consequences of removing the mandibular condyle on the growth of the maxilla and mandible in young rats. To assess the changes, axial and rostro-caudal radiographic views were taken of the fixed skull, and axial and lateral views of the hemimandibles; cephalometric measurements were taken to check the deviation from the midline using an angle formed by the midpoint between the tympanic bulla and the point between the incisors. To assess changes in the maxilla, measurements were taken between the tympanic bulla and the mesial root of the maxillary first molar, between the infla-orbital foramen and between the foramen and the incisal point. To assess changes in the mandible, the distance between the antegonal notch and the intersection of the distal face of the lower third molar with the ramus of the mandible was used to assess height, and the distance between the insertion of the incisor in the bone and the angular process was used to assess length. There was a significant deviation of the mandibular midline in the experimental group, a reduction in the height of the mandibular ramus, as well as its length.

There was a reduction in the length of the maxilla.

Takatsuka et al. (2005) analysed the influence of age and the degree of mandibular displacement on the repair of condylar fractures. They found that in young animals, fracture repair was complete regardless of the degree of displacement. In adult animals, repair was complete, but in the group with the greatest displacement there was a reduction in the height of the mandibular ramus with alterations in the fibrocartilage. They concluded that condylar deformities occur when the displacement of the fragments is greater.

Mandibular condylar cartilage differs from primary cartilage in the morphological organisation of chondrocytes and the response to biomechanical stress and humoral factors. This study describes the morphogenetics of bone morphogenetic protein 3 (Bmp3) in relation to types I, II and X collagen mRNA, in chondrocytes from rat mandibular condyle cartilage, femoral articular cartilage, augmented femoral growth plate cartilage and temporal cartilage. In bone remodelling, Bmp3 was verified in active osteoblast cells in post-fracture periosteum. Bmp3 was also found in periosteum layers of bone segments near the fracture site during healing. It is therefore suggested that Bmp3 in articular cartilage may be regulated by mechanical stress stimulation (ZHENG et al., 2005).

Teixeira, Teixeira and Luz (2006) carried out an experimental study to assess bone changes following condylar fractures during the growth period in young rats. The experimental group underwent a unilateral condyle fracture and the control-operated group only underwent surgical access. After three months, they were sacrificed and cephalometric assessments were carried out using axial views of the skull and lateral views of the hemimandibles. They concluded that the experimental fracture of the mandibular condyle during the growth period in rats induced degenerative changes in the condyle, as well as asymmetry of the mandible, affecting body height and also leading to consequences for the maxilla.

Porto, Vasconcelos and Silva Junior (2008) experimentally induced the development of ankylosis by removing the disc and injuring the TMJ of rats. There was weight loss in the 7-day period, with gain in the other periods. A histological study showed that there was no bone formation between the mandibular condyle and the temporal bone, but fibrous ankylosis developed in most of the animals.

2.3 Systemic conditions after fracture

However, studies have shown that, regardless of the surgical techniques used, weight loss decreases as the fracture heals (THALLER; REAVIE; DANILLER, 1990).

The changes in organic metabolism caused by trauma and surgery produce numerous problems related to protein, lipid and carbohydrate metabolism. Patients often have difficulty swallowing due to obstruction of the digestive tract. Of hospitalised patients, 30 to 50% have moderate or severe malnutrition as a result of either their primary disease or the therapy used to treat the underlying disease. In many circumstances, the primary disease leads to malnutrition, which in turn leads to altered healing, anaemia, reduced immunocompetence, reduced resistance to infection and septicaemia, which leads to worsening malnutrition, multiple organ failure and death. Facial fractures, especially mandibular fractures, cause patients to lose weight due to difficulty chewing, as well as moderate to severe malnutrition in 30 per cent of patients (MACHADO, 1993).

Rodrigues, Luz and Miori (1999) collected blood count data (erythrocyte, lymphocyte, monocyte, neutrophil and eosinophil counts, total leucocytes, haemoglobin, globular volume, mean globular volume) and blood biochemistry data (glucose, urea, creatinine, sodium and potassium) from patients with facial fractures. The authors found leucocytosis in 50% of the patients, neutrophilia in 68.7% and hyperglycemia in 26.9% of those analysed.

Kaplan, Hoard and Park (2001) carried out a study with 29 young patients, one group with mandibular fractures located at the angle of the mandible with immediate mobilisation and the other with two weeks of immobilisation with rigid internal fixation using 2mm titanium plates. All the fractures did not involve the alveoli, condyle, ramus or maxilla. Assessments were made after 6ª weeks, three and six months, checking for: pain, fracture repair with or without union, occlusion, trismus, wound condition, infection, dental hygiene and weight loss. There were no significant differences between the groups, only weight loss of 3.6 and 4.5 kg and trismus of 4.2 and 4.6 cm, respectively, were found to be significant.

Oliveira (2003) carried out an experimental study with adult rats (Lewis) to assess the influence of residronate sodium as an adjuvant in the treatment after 15 days of right tibial fractures, in nourished animals and those subjected to experimental malnutrition. Weight evolution, radiography, densitometry and histomorphometry of the bone callus and serum levels of calcium, phosphorus, alkaline phosphatase, total protein, albumin and osteocalcin were analysed. They observed weight loss in the high-protein diet groups after two weeks, which persisted until the end of the experiment, and a reduction in serum levels of calcium, alkaline phosphatase, total protein and albumin. They concluded that residronate had an influence on the fracture healing process, interfering positively with the animals' bone mineral density and the quality of the newly formed bone.

The increase in albumin values in fractures can be explained by the inflammatory process caused by the fracture itself, which increases circulating proteins, especially from the bone precursor matrix, and inflammatory mediators, especially collagen precursors (BORYS et al., 2004).

Luz and Rodrigues (2004) analysed variations in haemoglobin and haematocrit values at 1 week, 3 weeks and 6 weeks after orthognathic mandibular surgery. The authors detected a reduction in haemoglobin and haematocrit levels between the preoperative period and the 6-week postoperative period, with a slow recovery between the preoperative period and the postoperative period.

Dwyer et al. (2005) assessed 43 patients, with an average age of 28, with open fractures of the lower limbs over a 40-week period. Anthropometric, biochemical and haematological parameters were used to analyse their relationship with soft tissue healing after trauma. In the initial phase, twenty-one patients were found to be malnourished. A diet and good food intake reduced malnutrition, leaving only 13 malnourished patients after 40 weeks. Among the parameters used to determine nutritional status, biochemical tests were used to determine creatinine, serum albumin, serum transferrin and total lymphocyte count. They found that soft tissue healing took less time when the creatinine index was normal and was delayed when the serum albumin level was lower.

Kommenou et al. (2005) analysed the correlation between alkaline phosphatase activity, calcium and phosphorus with the repair of closed long bone fractures in dogs. Alkaline phosphatase activity, calcium and phosphorus concentrations were determined. For the division into groups, the progression of bone callus formation was taken into account, with group A developing medium-sized calluses with repair in 2 months. Group B had callus hypertrophy and delayed bone union for 3 to 5 months. Group C, with a slow process and reduced callus formation without stump union within two months. Alkaline phosphatase in groups A and B had a maximum increase at 10 days. Group A returned to normal at 60 days and group B at 3 to 5 months. Group C showed no significant changes. Phosphorus and calcium showed changes proportionally inverse to those of alkaline phosphatase. They concluded that the serial determination of alkaline phosphatase activities during fracture repair can help to assess the process of bone neoformation, collaborating in the appropriate choice of clinical intervention.

Seebeck et al. (2005) evaluated the correlation between serological parameters during the development of bone callus in tibial fractures in sheep. There was bone callus formation and all serological parameters showed wide individual variations in the fractured and control group. The level of acid phosphatase was reduced during bone callus formation and the level of type II procollagen was increased. Osteocalcin showed a significant decrease. There was an increase in calcium, alkaline phosphatase showed a reduction in bone-specific alkaline phosphatase as well as resistant alkaline phosphatase. However, the difference in total alkaline phosphatase serology and the bone-specific alkaline phosphatase / total alkaline phosphatase ratio between the groups was not significant.

Hughes et al. (2006) carried out an experimental study to verify the effects of a protein and amino acid diet on muscle and bone healing after a femur fracture in adult rats. There was a control group and a group on a low-protein diet (6% protein). After the fracture, they were subdivided into groups with a 6% protein diet, 15% protein and 30% protein associated with amino acids. The femur was assessed by radiography, callus histomorphometry and torsion test. The quadriceps muscles were assessed for total mass and total protein content. From the results, the 30% protein group after 6 weeks showed an increase in albumin, body and muscle mass, total protein in the muscle and bone density when compared to the 6% protein groups. When analysing the muscle, the biometric tests of the femur showed no significant difference. They concluded that supplementary amino acid diets in malnourished animals had anabolic effects on bone repair, body and muscle mass.

Miller et al. (2006) studied a group of 68 hospitalised patients, with an average age of 70, classified as undernourished, with a lower limb fracture, 50% of whom had cognitive impairment. These patients were given an energy and protein diet for 3 to 5 days, 6 days after the trauma. Protein requirements were calculated as 1g/Kg/day. They found that the patients, including those with cognitive impairment, did not reach their energy and protein requirements with the enriched diet alone.

2.4 Effects of malnutrition

According to the World Health Organisation (WHO, 1962), malnutrition is a condition of protein-calorie deficiency that includes severe forms such as marasmus (insufficient calorie supply) and Kwashiorkor (severe protein deprivation), as well as phases and moderate forms.

It is estimated that malnutrition affects between half and two thirds of the world's population. The prevalence of infectious diseases in areas where hunger is endemic makes the situation even more serious, since resistance to infection in these populations is much lower. As a result, the severity of infectious processes and mortality are higher in the malnourished population, especially in children, who are the age group most vulnerable to their effects (YUNES, 1976).

The importance of collagen synthesis in the calcification process has been reported. In this study, Nakamoto and Miller (1979a) analysed collagen synthesis, calcium deposition and calcium half-life in the mandible and long bones of newborn rats fed a hypoprotein diet (6%) and a control group (25%). They observed interference in collagen synthesis in the long bones of animals with protein malnutrition. However, calcium absorption occurs in parallel with bone matrix formation and was equivalent in both groups. The half-life of calcium in the long bones and mandible in both groups was 72 hours, differing only in the long bones of the control group, with a half-life of 100 hours.

Nakamoto and Miller (1979b) studied the influence of a hypoprotein diet on the mandibular development of newborn rats, creating an experimental model of moderate calorific-protein malnutrition. The authors compared mandibular development with that of the long bones (femur and tibia) in terms of weight and the amount of calcium, DNA and RNA and proteins. They found that the weight of the mandibles of the malnourished rats was significantly reduced compared to the control, but this did not affect mandibular growth on average. There was a greater weight reduction in the long bones compared to the mandible, which suggests that the mandibular bone must have some compensatory mechanism for protein deprivation. The mandibles showed satisfactory calcification compared to the long bones, as well as a quantity of proteins very close to the control. The amount of DNA and RNA in the protein-deprived mandibles substantially exceeded that of the control.

In another experiment, Nakamoto, Porter and Winkler (1983) verified the effects of protein malnutrition on the metabolism of growth centres in the mandibles and long bones of newborn rats with a gestational history of malnutrition. These animals showed a reduction in mandibular and long bone weight and a greater amount of cells and calcium in the mandible compared to the control. These quantities were not altered in the long bones, which led the authors to conclude that bone metabolism in the different growth centres subjected to nutritional stress shows different behaviour when considering the mandible and long bones.

Alippi et al. (1984) carried out an experimental study on rats to check the effects of a protein-free diet on the skeletal development of rat jaws. One group was given a protein-free diet and the other a 20% casein diet. Linear measurements of the mandible were taken to assess growth. They found significant differences between the different measurements. As a result, they found that when the mandible was considered as a whole, the effect of the diets was different. The average mandibular weight and thickness was greater in the control group. They concluded that the rats on the protein-free diet had altered mandibular bone proportions with bone deformities.

Jones, Simson and Friedman (1984) in a study of rats that suffered intrauterine malnutrition observed hyperphagia and the accumulation of body fat in early adulthood, suggesting that obesity could occur as a sequel to previous energy-protein malnutrition. This sequel would occur due to a modification in the regulation of the central nervous system in the sense of prioritising the accumulation of body fat in order to promote a positive energy balance when food availability increased.

Miwa et al. (1989), studying rat foetuses subjected to protein restriction, found that the animals' mandibles had higher protein and hexosamine levels than the calvaria and lower calcium levels in both bones. The mandible showed lower amounts of low molecular weight proteoglycan subunits, which were dissociated. The authors concluded that the insufficient degradation of proteoglycans seems to be the reason for the poor mineralisation observed in the bones of the foetus.

Rodrigues and Zucas (1991) carried out a study to verify the effect of energy and/or protein malnutrition on the evolution of bone callus formation in fractures of the left humerus of Wistar rats in the growth and adult phases. The protein sources were soya protein and skimmed milk powder. Energy malnutrition was achieved by eating a diet equivalent to 60 per cent of the group ad libitum. Radiographic observations of the fractured bones did not consistently show the influence of malnutrition on the evolution of bone callus formation. The young rats showed evidence of faster bone regeneration and there was a delay in the evolution of bone callus in the adult animals whose diet was hypoproteinised.

Guarniero et al. (1992) carried out a study to verify the effects of protein malnutrition on the repair of tibial fractures in rats. Weight variation, fracture healing by radiography of the bone callus, macroscopic assessment of the mechanical strength of the bone callus and histological examination were analysed. They concluded that in the normal diet and renourished groups, there was normal bone callus formation, with regular tissue, and in the protein malnutrition groups there was fibrous tissue formation with less bone tissue formation.

Konno et al. (1993) evaluated the effect of a high-protein diet or diet restriction on the immune system of rats at different ages. They observed a reduction in the thymus gland and a reduction in T lymphocyte cells in animals fed a high-protein diet. The depressive effect on the immune system was greater in young mice than in adults. The results suggested that the function of the thymus is altered in the face of protein deficiency, that a balanced diet is necessary for immune maturation at an early stage of life, that immune functions are preserved in the elderly, and that animals with increased immune functions are more resistant to malnutrition.

According to UNICEF (1994), for every one child who dies from energy-protein malnutrition, another six survive in hunger and disease. In South America, a study of childhood mortality revealed that energy-protein malnutrition and/or low birth weight were present in 57 per cent of deaths in children under 5.

The state of malnutrition can be considered primary: when there is inadequate intake of nutrients due to a lack of food or an inappropriate ratio of food, secondary: resulting from inadequate intake of nutrients as a sequel to diseases that lead to problems with ingestion, chewing, swallowing, digestion and absorption, and tertiary: resulting from the administration of intravenous solutions in a hospital environment, having an iatrogenic characteristic (AUN, 1997).

Chandra (1999, 2002) considered that diet and immunity are interrelated, as nutritional deficiencies impair the immune response and often result in serious infections resulting in increased mortality, especially in children. Protein-energy malnutrition results in a reduction in the number and function of T lymphocytes, phagocytic cells and in the secretory immunoglobulin A antibody response. The use of supplements stimulates immunity and can result in a reduction in infections, especially in the elderly, low birth weight newborns and malnourished patients in hospital.

Costa et al. (2000) carried out an experimental study to assess the effectiveness of molasses supplementation in the diet of normal and depleted rats. Groups with: casein with 10.14% protein, casein molasses with 10.14% protein and molasses at 12.50% depleted control and depleted molasses without protein. Feed and weight were monitored to calculate the feed efficiency ratio (FEC). For the biochemical analysis, 2ml of blood was taken by cardiac puncture and placed in tubes containing EDTA anticoagulant to determine haemoglobin. They found that feed consumption in the molasses-supplemented group was higher (9 per cent) than in the control group, but there was no significant increase in weight, although CEA was lower in this group compared to the casein-supplemented group without depletion. As a result, they observed that there was no significant increase in the average haemoglobin concentration.

Campos (2001) carried out a study on the effect of the ossein hydroxy apatite complex on the healing of closed fractures of the middle third of the left tibia in rats on protein malnutrition. After 4 weeks, radiographic, planimetric, densitometric, weight control, histological and histomorphometric studies were carried out, as well as biochemical analyses - calcium, phosphorus, alkaline phosphatase, total proteins, albumin and osteocalcin. It was concluded that the ossein-hydroxyapatite complex did not interfere with the formation of bone callus in either the nourished or malnourished animals, although it did interfere with some results, such as albumin and alkaline phosphatase levels, planimetry and animal weight.

Day and DeHeer (2001) carried out an experimental study on rats with a hypoprotein diet (6% protein) and a conventional diet (20% protein) in femur fractures and applied mechanical resistance tests to assess bone healing. They observed that animals with protein malnutrition produced calluses composed of fibrous tissue, with reduced periosteum and external calluses. Based on mechanical tests, the calluses of malnourished animals showed reduced strength and hardness when compared to the other groups. They concluded that protein deprivation has a detrimental effect on fracture healing. Identifying the state of protein malnutrition and reversing it could result in an improved outcome and probably a clinical improvement in malnourished patients.

Pallaro, Roux and Slobodianik (2001) studied the effect of a low-protein diet (6.5% protein) on cell proliferation and thymus maturation in young rats. They analysed food intake, body weight, thymus weight, total number of thymocytes and the percentage of phenotypic thymocyte antigen. The results indicated that consumption of a low-protein diet causes thymus atrophy in growing rats, with a significant reduction in total T lymphocyte cells, concomitant with an increase in immature thymocytes. They concluded that the hypoprotein diet is a factor that limits the chemical reactions of intrathymic cells, probably related to the need for specific amino acids for a more favourable immune response.

SanfiAna et al. (2001) experimentally studied the presence of retroperitoneal fat in malnourished adult rats. The experimental group had a 14.8 per cent reduction in body weight and an increase in average peritoneal fat of 8.7, compared to the control group with 7.43. They suggested that in the experimental group, despite the weight reduction shown, they actually gained weight due to the accumulation of fat from the excess carbohydrate present in the low-protein diet offered, which caused a change in body composition with an increase in fat in relation to the lean mass of the malnourished animals.

Laing and Fraser (2002) examined the possible effects of nutritional deficiency on the characteristics of protein transport in plasma by vitamin D and on metabolism (vitamin D with protein) in growing rats. A diet deficient in protein and energy can reduce the concentration of protein and vitamin D in the circulation. However, they observed that vitamin D and plasma protein may not be affected by a diet deficient in calcium. None of the dietary factors examined had an influence. They observed that protein-deficient rats seem to have difficulty maintaining adequate calcium concentrations in the circulation. The introduction of a high-protein, high-energy diet may constitute a new mechanism that could help explain the observed association between malnutrition and the development of metabolic bone diseases, and cellular assessment of vitamin D changes associated with protein could be a tool.

Araújo et al. (2003 a,b) used the same malnutrition methodology in adult rats to check its effects on the myenteric plexus of the descending colon. They found an 11.84 per cent reduction in the body weight of animals submitted to a diet with a protein content of 8 per cent and restriction of B vitamins and suggest that these biomolecules, in balanced quantities, are fundamental for weight gain, outweighing the importance of starch, which was present in excess in the diet used. They suggested that, despite the dilution of protein and vitamin levels through the addition of starch, the concentrations that remained may have been sufficient to prevent clinical manifestations of malnutrition.

Guarniero et al. (2003) studied the influence of protein nutrition on the healing of left tibia fractures in rats. Clinical, biochemical, radiographic, densitometric and hy- tomorphometric measurements were used to assess the results. The results showed a marked decrease in weight with the high-protein diet, as well as a drop in total protein and albumin levels when compared to the normal and high-protein diet groups. In terms of fracture healing, the high-protein diet group had one case of non-fracture healing and the rest had intermediate healing. In quantitative measurements, the bone callus was larger in area and more resistant in the animals on the high-protein diet. The greater resistance may be due to the greater quantity of organic structures and not to the increased concentration of minerals. It was concluded that the high-protein diet altered bone healing, producing a larger and more resistant callus, but did not alter the quality in terms of calcium concentration or the percentage of bone tissue quantity.

Zanin (2003) evaluated the effect of protein and B vitamin deficiency on the myenteric plexus of the duodenum in adult rats. The control group was given unrestricted commercial feed with B vitamins and a 22% protein content for 120 days. The experimental group was given a 120-day diet with a protein content of 8% obtained by adding starch and without vitamin supplementation. At the end of the experiment, the animals showed weight loss, a reduction in total protein and albumin. The blood count was unchanged for both groups. The NADH-diaphoresis technique showed that there was a difference in the size of neurons, little evidence of neurons and tertiary meshes in the experimental group. There was also a reduction in the number and density of neurons. However, there was no statistically significant difference.

Santos et al. (2004) assessed testosterone concentration, sexual behaviour and the level of androgen receptor protein in adult male rats submitted to a hypoprotein and energy diet for 30 days. They divided them into a control group with a standard diet containing 23% protein, a protein-restricted group with a diet containing 8% protein and added vitamins and minerals prepared in the laboratory, and an energy-restricted group consuming 50% of the standard diet. As a result, they found that the experimental group showed changes in androgen receptor protein levels, testosterone concentration and sexual behaviour.

The growth and development of the human skeleton requires an adequate supply of many different nutritional factors. Classic nutritional deficiencies are associated with dwarfism (energy, protein and zinc), rickets (vitamin D) and other bone abnormalities (Cu, Zn, vitamin C). Recently, it has become clear that nutrition plays a role in bone growth and in preventing classic deficiencies, which can reduce the risk of osteoporosis. It is suggested that they are influenced by the pattern of growth during the intrauterine period, childhood and adolescence. Calcium, vitamin D, protein and phosphorus are found in dairy products, fruit and vegetables. However, it is not possible to establish a reference value for the diet with the best supply for bone formation. It is known that calcium intake, optimising the amount of vitamin D through exposure to the sun, supplementary diet when necessary, physical activity, adequate weight, restricting salt intake and consuming plenty of fruit and vegetables are adequate measures for bone growth and development (PRENTICE et al., 2006).

Prestes-Carneiro et al. (2006) assessed the effect of protein malnutrition on growth using haematological parameters and macrophage function in adult rats. They compared animals and their offspring that were fed a 9.5 per cent protein hypoprotein diet or a 23 per cent protein diet for the first 12 days of breastfeeding. At 80 days of age, the function of macrophages residing in the peritoneum was assessed, as well as the leucocyte count and red blood cell count. There was a drop in the red series of the blood count, but no significant difference in leucocytes between the groups. They observed that the group given a low-protein diet during breastfeeding had alterations in macrophage function, which was not restored after eating a normal diet, with a significant reduction in pup growth.

Hoffman et al. (2007) studied the variation in central fat distribution between children with growth retardation and children with normal growth over four years in a favela community in São Paulo. To do this, they carried out measurements of fat mass and fat distribution. During the follow-up, they found that the children with growth retardation had lower weights and lower fat mass ratios when compared to the control group. Linear regression analyses were used to determine that children with growth retardation had an increase in the percentage of fat mass in the abdomen with significant changes in its limit. They concluded that children with growth retardation are prone to depositing fat centrally when they are entering puberty, which is a risk factor for chronic diseases. These results may explain part of the association between early growth retardation and later risks for metabolic diseases. In Brazil, malnutrition in urban children and adolescents is characterised by poor linear growth associated or not with reduced body weight and increased fat deposits in the abdomen.

Pompeo (2007) reported that successful treatment for patients with healing wounds and protein malnutrition is critical. To ascertain the causes of poor nutrition, a one-year prospective study was carried out with enterally fed patients with and without wounds. Initially, 11 per cent of the injured and 21 per cent of those without injuries had normal prealbumin levels. With the addition of a high-protein diet, 42 per cent of patients with injuries and 46 per cent without injuries showed an increase in prealbumin levels. The average amount of protein given to patients with wounds was 1.85g/Kg/day, and for the group without wounds it was 1.47g/Kg/day. He concluded that patients with wounds require more protein and that the likelihood of normalising the protein supply in enterally-fed patients is small, as the risk of complications arising from supplies lower than the protein requirement in the enteral diet is high, as is the risk of offering higher supplies.

Nakajima et al. (2008) evaluated the effects of protein malnutrition on the intestinal wall by measuring the rupture force and tissue collagen in the ileum and distal colon of rats. The rats were divided into two groups, one with a normal diet and the other with a hypoprotein diet containing 2% casein. Body weight, albumin, tissue hydroxyproline, hydroproline ratio, tissue protein and rupture force were assessed in the ileal and colonic segments of the animals. Body weight and serum albumin values were lower at all times in the malnourished group. They observed that the rupture force of the ileal segment and distal colon was lower in the malnourished animals. The loss of mechanical resistance was greater in the distal colon segment than in the ileal segment, probably due to the lower concentration of tissue collagen in the distal colon. They concluded that protein malnutrition induces a decrease in resistance in the ileum and distal colon associated with a decrease in tissue collagen in the intestinal wall.

2.5 Malnutrition indicators

Campbell (1963) described that the control of feed efficiency is the result of the values obtained from the weekly feed supply and consumption with the initial and final weight values of the experiment, obtaining the Feed Efficiency Coefficient (FEC).

The coefficient of feed efficiency (CEA) evaluates the body weight gain of an animal fed a specific diet during a test period. This index assesses the efficiency with which the diet promotes body weight gain, so it evaluates the feed as a whole and not just the efficiency and quality of the proteins. If a diet is nutritionally balanced, the values found for CEA will be high when compared to standard protein (PELLET and YOUNG, 1980; SGARBIERI, 1987).

In order to assess nutritional status, it is necessary to determine a profile of different parameters. This profile incorporates various tests, measurements and derived parameters, established and adapted for clinical use in identifying the state of malnutrition from standards for nutritional support and assessing the response to nutritional therapy. Biochemical analysis can be applied to assess nutritional status, such as determining values for: creatinine, serum albumin, serum transferrin, total lymphocyte count, as well as immunological assessment (DE LEEUW; VANDEWOUDE; VAN ELST, 1981).

Kergoat et al. (1987) carried out a study to verify the serum markers that most determine protein-energy conditions of malnutrition in elderly patients. They found that only the classic serum indices and retinol-bound protein can predict malnutrition. They stated that creatinine, urea, complement C3 and prealbumin and, above all, serum carotene can be included in malnourished elderly patients.

A patient's nutritional status is an important factor to assess in oral and maxillofacial surgery. The success or failure of the outcome will depend on the patient's nutritional status to promote a better response from the immune deficiency mechanism, avoiding susceptibility to infection, as well as adequate healing. During the initial clinical examination, you should be on the lookout for signs and symptoms of nutritional deficiency. If a nutritional deficiency is present, it can be treated pre-surgery with a balanced diet and supplements, as well as maintaining adequate protein intake post-surgery (CHIDYLLO; CHIDYLLO, 1989).

Malnutrition is known as one of the main medical problems, especially in developing countries. The presence of protein-calorie malnutrition results in a significant increase in the incidence of mortality and morbidity in the hospital environment. The application of nutritional status assessment techniques has revealed, for example, that around 50 per cent of patients admitted to different in-hospital services have varying degrees of malnutrition. Many of the patients who develop protein-energy malnutrition are admitted with a history of weight loss, resulting from anorexia and increased catabolism associated with the catabolic trauma of surgery. Protein loss reduces resistance to infection, prevents tissue repair and interferes with the synthesis of enzymes and plasma proteins (VANNUCCHI; UNAMUNO; MARCHINI, 1996).

Nóbrega (1998) stated that in the pre-clinical period of malnutrition there are already biochemical changes that induce functional anatomical alterations, but the speed of the alterations depends on the organic reserves of nutrients and the adaptive metabolic changes that try to make up for the deficiency. He reports that when the period of malnutrition is not long and is followed by a return to a protein diet, there is a possibility of morphofunctional reversal. However, the earlier and longer the deficiency state, the more serious the injuries and the lower the chances of recovery. The absence of structural changes in the animals in the experimental group suggests that the period used here was not enough to promote them.

Vitamin D deficiency has been observed in elderly patients. In this study, they found significant differences in vitamin D levels in women with hip fractures, with no medical history of secondary comorbidity. They found that women with osteoporosis (17% of patients hospitalised with hip fracture) were vitamin D deficient. They also found a decrease in albumin in women with hip fractures, reflecting a poor nutritional state and consequent vitamin D deficiency. The external protection of the hip, the importance of good nutrition enriched with vitamin D in postmenopausal women can reduce the rate of fractures (LÊ BOFF et al., 2000).

Ribeiro Passos De Oliveira et al. (2001) evaluated the nutritional value of cassava flour enriched with bioproteins associated with commonly consumed mixtures in Wistar rats. They measured weight gain and food intake. The CEA (coefficient of food efficiency) was evaluated. The data suggested that cassava flour enriched with bioproteins improves the food mixture.

Sheiham et al. (2001) carried out a study to verify the relationship between dental and nutritional status in elderly patients. An examination of dental conditions, interviews, diet control and blood and urine analyses were carried out. Edentulous patients had lower food intake compared to dentate patients. Dentate patients with 21 or more teeth consumed more. There was no significant difference in the haematological analysis.

Stark, Bennet and Stone (2002) verified the relationship between childhood fractures and poverty and assessed levels of deprivation to compare health status in social areas that differed in this association. Children in deprived areas had a significantly higher rate of fractures than those in affluent areas. This finding correlates with previous reports of increased mortality from disease. This study is useful for monitoring the effects of programmes targeting the underserved and in urban regeneration and health promotion projects.

Bone morphological changes caused by malnutrition in animals include a reduction in size and a delay in the appearance of ossification centres in relation to gestational age. Boldrini (2003) assessed the effects of pre- and post-natal protein malnutrition and post-natal renutrition on the craniofacial growth of wistar rats by means of cephalometric, linear and angular, morphoquantitative and ultrastructural analyses. The study used young males and females, and after mating, the females were separated into groups: nourished, with a protein diet (20% casein), and malnourished with a hypoprotein diet (5% casein). After 21 days of life, the male chicks were separated into their respective groups and diets. After 42 days, they were subjected to different techniques. In the malnourished group, it was found that linear measurements were affected by malnutrition, with smaller measurements, alterations characteristic of a delay in normal development and a significant decrease in the number of cells in mitosis with malnutrition.

Ortega-Flores et al. (2003) analysed the protein quality of dehydrated cassava leaves in a 25-day biological trial on rats. At the end, the carcasses and faeces were analysed. Food consumption and animal weight were monitored. The indices used were Feed Efficiency Ratio (FEC), Net Protein

Ratio (NPR), True Digestibility Coefficient (CDv), True Net Protein Utilisation (NPV) and Biological Value (BV). They concluded that the protein quality of dehydrated cassava leaf was inferior to casein.

Enteropathies with protein loss were diagnosed in two dogs that presented with diarrhoea and weight loss. Biochemical tests on both revealed low concentrations of albumin, calcium and ionised calcium. Both had high plasma parathyroid hormone concentrations and low serum hydroxyvitamin D concentrations. They considered that enteropathies with protein loss may reduce the intestinal absorption of vitamin D with a lower concentration of calcium in the plasma, and low concentrations of albumin and calcium were detected (MELLANBY et al., 2005).

The loss of teeth can lead to a reduction in food intake, making the diet deficient. The risk of malnutrition can be associated with various factors, including prosthetic conditions. Oliveira; Frigerio (2005) carried out a comparative study between conventional total prostheses (CTP) and implant-retained mu- co-supported prostheses (RMSP). There were two groups of patients of both genders with bimaxillary total edentulism, one group rehabilitated with CTP and the other with mandibular and maxillary CTP. A clinical examination, interview and nutritional test, occlusion, vertical dimension (VD), masticatory ability and satisfaction with the prostheses were carried out. They concluded that patients with CTP had a higher risk of malnutrition and lower chewing ability. The assessment of occlusion and OVD, and the degree of satisfaction with the prostheses was satisfactory for both groups.

CHAPTER 3

PROPOSAL

The aim of this study was to assess repair and malnutrition indicators in rats submitted to mandibular condyle fracture and protein malnutrition.

CHAPTER 4

MATERIALS AND METHODS

4.1 Animals

We used 45 three-month-old adult male Wistar rats from the Central Animal Facility of the Institute of Bio-Medical Sciences (ICB) of the University of São Paulo, which were kept in individual cages in the Experimental Laboratory of the Department of Oral and Maxillofacial Surgery and Traumatology of the School of Dentistry of the University of São Paulo. The animals were handled in accordance with the ethical principles proposed by the Brazilian College of Animal Experimentation. The research was approved by the Research Ethics Committee of the University of São Paulo School of Dentistry, under Protocol No. 08/05 (Annex A).

The animals were divided into three groups, distributed as follows: **F -Fractured** -15 animals submitted to a unilateral condylar fracture on the right side with rotation.

- no change in diet, comprising granulated commercial rodent food, with fine granulation in the first week and normal granulation up to 90 days, and water ad libitum.

FD -Fractured Malnourished -15 animals submitted to a unilateral condylar fracture on the right side with rotation, and with a change in diet:

- with previous protein malnutrition for 30 days pre-surgery, receiving a hypoprotein diet - 8% protein and water ad libitum. This group comprised individuals who were notably malnourished due to nutritional changes, had undergone a fracture and remained malnourished throughout the experiment.

D - Malnourished - 15 animals.

- with previous protein malnutrition, receiving a hypoprotein diet - 8% protein and water ad libitum. This group comprised individuals who were notably malnourished due to nutritional changes, had not undergone surgery and remained malnourished throughout the experiment.

The animals were sacrificed at 24 hours, 7 days, 15 days, 30 days and 90 days, comprising three animals for each period in each group.

At the same time, a negative control group (NC) was set up with five animals weighing 320 grams without being subjected to malnutrition or fracture. They were sacrificed after 90 days and their blood was taken for biochemical tests and leucograms.

The animals with no change in diet were fed commercial pelleted rodent food (Labina, Agribrands Purina) with a 23 per cent protein content, vitamins and minerals (Appendix B).

The animals with altered diets were fed special prepared granulated feed. Protein malnutrition was induced by administering a ration with only 8% protein (Appendix B). This feed was manipulated with a mixture of corn starch and water, as described in Santos et al. (2004). The vitamin and mineral content was also compensated for using a controlled mixture of these (Appendices C, D and E).

The procedure for making one kilogram of hypoprotein feed, according to Santos et al. (2004) involved the following steps:

weighing 348 g of commercial crushed rodent food (Labina®, Purina do Brasil);

- weighing 591 g of cornstarch;
- weighing 26 g of salts (Pre-Mix Mineral AIN-93M, Rhoster Ind. Com. Ltda., Brazil) (Appendix D);
- mixture of the above items with 32 ml of soya oil, mixed beforehand with 26g of vitamins (Appendix E);
- adding water until a dough is obtained;
- making pellets by hand;
- cooking them in an oven at 180°C until they become hard, for approximately 2 hours.

Around 24kg of feed was used to induce malnutrition in the animals. The amount of water ingested (in ml) and feed ingested (in grams) was documented weekly, as well as the amount of water left over and the amount of feed wasted.

Food Efficiency Ratio

The coefficient of feed efficiency (CEA) was calculated for each animal in all the experimental groups. The feed efficiency ratio is the ratio of animal weight to feed consumption. It was calculated on the basis of the average weekly feed consumption, the difference between the feed offered and the residual feed, and the weight of the animal at the start of the experiment, at the time of the fracture and at sacrifice. For the fractured group, the average feed consumption was calculated from the day of the fracture. For the malnourished group, the average feed consumption during the malnutrition period was calculated, taking into account the previous four weeks (30 days) for all experimental periods. For the malnourished fractured group, the feed efficiency ratio was calculated based on the previous four weeks of malnutrition, plus the experimental period following the fracture (Appendix F).

Body weight

All the animals were weighed at the start of the experiment, pre-surgery and at sacrifice, using a standardised digital scale (Coleman, Brazil). For the fractured group, the weight at the beginning and on the day of the fracture was the same, since time zero of the experiment for this group coincided with the day of the fracture, since the animals had not previously been malnourished. In the malnourished group, there is no weight value on the day of the fracture, as the animals in this group were not subjected to the fracture.

Surgical procedure

The animals underwent general anaesthesia using xylidine dihydrotizanine hydrochloride (Rompum, Bayer) at a dose of 0.8 mg/kg body weight and ketamine hydrochloride (Francotar, Francodex) at a dose of 10 mg/100g body weight, both drugs applied intraperitoneally.

Subsequently, the right pre-auricular region was trichotomised, followed by antisepsis with polyvinylpyrrolidone-iodine solution. Access to the condyle was obtained through a 10 mm pre-auricular incision, followed by dissection of the masseter muscle below the zygomatic arch, exposing the condylar process. This process was fractured using mosquito forceps, after which the condylar head was rotated medially, keeping the articular surfaces intact (LUZ; ARAÚJO, 2001). The surgical procedure was completed by suturing the planes with 4.0 monofilament nylon thread. The left side of each animal was kept as a fracture control, without any intervention.

The animals undergoing surgery received prophylactic antibiotic administration with benzathine benzylpenicillin (Benzetacil 1,200,000 UI, Fontoura-Wyeth S.A.) at a dose of 0.01 mg/100g body weight and potassium and procaine penicillin G (Despacilin 400,000 UI, Bristol-Myers Squibb) at a dose of 0.02 ml/100g body weight, intraperitoneally. After the end of the experimental periods, the animals were sacrificed with a lethal dose of general anaesthetic. The temporomandibular joints were obtained and decalcified for subsequent microscopic morphological analysis.

4.2 Laboratory tests

Blood was taken from the animals at the end of the experiment to carry out biochemical blood tests such as: total proteins, serum albumin, serum calcium, alkaline phosphatase, serum iron and creatinine, as well as haematological tests represented by the leucogram. These tests were used to detect systemic alterations that could justify a possible malnutrition due to the difficulty in feeding the animals or the diet established for each group, as well as the inflammatory condition established during the repair process. Biochemical and haematological tests were carried out manually.

Standardisation of blood collection and processing

2ml of the animal's blood was collected by cardiac puncture at the time of sacrifice during the established experimental periods. A small part of the blood collected was placed in a vacuum tube with liquid EDTA, and the rest was poured into a dry vacuum tube. After collection, the blood was immediately swabbed and the global leucocyte count was performed manually in a Neubauer chamber (Loptik®, Labor). The blood inserted into the dry tube was centrifuged (Coleman, mod. 90-1) at 300 rpm for 10 minutes. The serum obtained was then removed using a pipette, placed in an Eppendorf tube and stored in a refrigerator at -7°C.

The material was subjected to the reaction using the respective reagent and standard kits (Labtest® São Paulo, Brazil), in accordance with the manufacturer's standards. The reaction was quantified using a previously calibrated spectrophotometer (Coleman, mod. 35D). A previous calibration period for the animal samples was necessary.

Biochemical tests

The reference values for the animals' biochemical blood tests were obtained from the values of the negative control and those reported by Mitruka and Rawnsley (1977) (Appendix H).

Leucogram

The average value of the global leucocyte count found in the negative control animals was 3.6 ± 1.5x103/mm3 and the reference value for total leucocytes was 3.3 to 8.3x103/mm3 (SANDERSON; PHILIPS, 1981).

The percentage distribution of leucocytes in the individual count of adult male rats

(SANDERSON; PHILIPS, 1981), the negative control and the reference values (MITRUKA; RAWNSLEY, 1977) are shown in Appendix I and J.

4.3 Cephalometric measurements using radiographs

For the radiographic examination, an odontological X-ray machine (Spectro II, Dabi-Atlante, Ribeirão Preto, Brazil) was used at 56 kV, 10 mA and 0.4 seconds, and periapical radiographic film (Kodak-Ektaspeed, Eastman Kodak Co, USA). The animals' heads were held in a horizontal plane 40 centimetres away from the focus and submitted to an axial view of the skull.

A computerised system was used to obtain the measurements, which were taken at the Laboratory of Information Technology Dedicated to Dentistry (LIDO), using an IBM-PC microcomputer (International Business Machines corporation, USA). The images were acquired and processed using the electronic retina of the Fotovix II (Tamron Co., Japan) and transferred to the microcomputer using the Iris 16 card (marketed by the Microimagem company). They were observed on the Sony Trinitron monitor (Sony Co., Japan) and digitised using the Image-Lab software (Softium Informática, São Paulo, Brazil). calibrated in millimetres, which allowed linear measurements of reproducible points to be made.

In the axial view of the skull, a line was drawn immediately anterior to the tympanic bulla on the right and left sides, and the median point was determined. Then, based on the point between the upper incisors (PI) and lower incisors (PI'), the angle formed was measured, known as angle Â, allowing the deviation from the midline between the maxilla and mandible to be quantified (Figure 4.1).

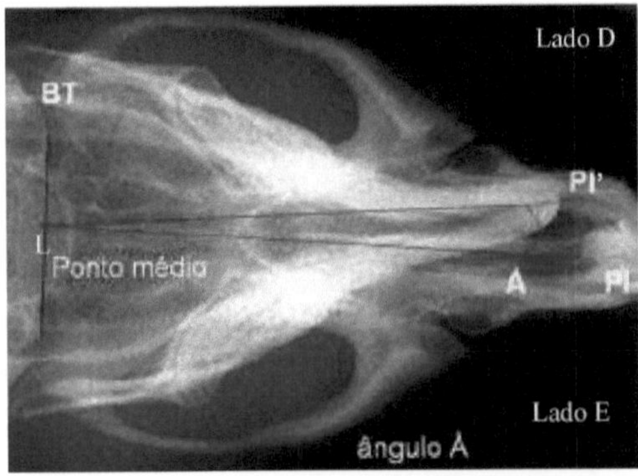

Figura 4.1 - Determination of the Angle Â in the axial view of the skull. BT = tympanic bulla (right and left) midpoint; PI = incisal point between the upper incisors and PI' = incisal point between the lower incisors.

In the axial view of the skull, the distance between the tympanic bulla and the infraorbital foramen (BT-FI) and the distance between the infraorbital foramen and the incisal point (FI-PI) were measured in the maxilla (Figure 4.2).

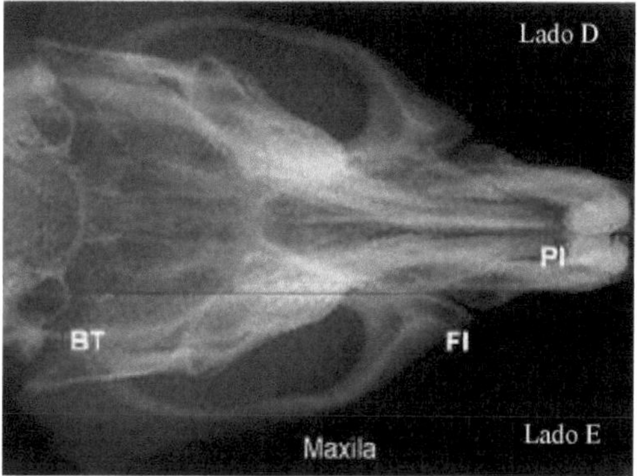

Figura 4.2 Measurements of the maxilla in the axial view of the skull.
PI = incisal point; FI = infraorbital foramen; BT = tympanic bulla

In the axial view of the skull, the distance between the angular process and the insertion of the incisor (PA-II) and the angular process and the incisal point (PA-PF) were measured on the mandible (Figure 4.3).

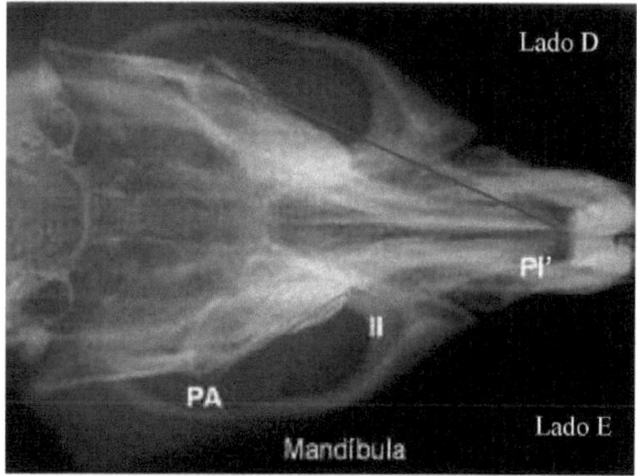

Figure 4.3. Measurements of the mandible in the axial view of the skull. PI' = incisal point; PA = angular process; II = incisor insertion

4.4 Histological study of the TMJs

Standardisation of necropsy and decalcification **of TMJs**

The animals' heads were removed and fixed in 10% formalin for a week. After this period,

they were cut in half in the sagittal plane with a surgical microsaw (Stryker®, Michigan, USA) and kept under fixation for a further two days. The right (fractured) side was washed with running water for 20 minutes and then placed in a 10% EDTA solution, pH 7.4. The solution was changed every two days for two months. 10 hemi-heads were standardised for working
together, carrying out 6 microwave cycles three times a week at a maximum temperature of 35°C. 140 cycles of 15 minutes each were carried out, totalling 27 hours of processing. The EDTA solution was changed every four cycles. Subsequently, the material was embedded and blocked in paraffin. Serial sections of four pm were stained in haematoxylin-eosin according to the routine technique.

Histological analysis

The TMJs were routinely processed for observation under an ordinary optical microscope, based on frontal sections. The specimens were assessed for the formation of bone trabeculae and cartilaginous tissue, the differentiation of osteoblastic and osteoclastic cells and the presence of inflammatory exudate. The characteristics and topography of the articular surfaces of the condyle and mandibular fossa, as well as the articular disc, were also assessed.

4.5 Statistical analysis

The values obtained were tabulated and statistically processed using the SPSS (Statistical Package for Social Sciences) programme in its version 13.0 for Windows. To compare the three groups studied, the Analysis of Variance (ANOVA) was applied, controlled by Levene's Test for Equality of Variances, in order to check for possible differences between the three groups studied, when compared concomitantly. For the variables of interest in which a statistically significant difference was found, the Tukey or Dunnet test was applied, as appropriate, to identify which groups differed from one another. The *Friedman* test was applied to the comparison between moments, by group, in order to check for possible differences between the observation moments, when compared concomitantly, in each group, for the variables of interest. For each block of variables in which a statistically significant difference was found, the *Student's t-test for paired data* was then applied to identify which moments differed from the others. A significance level of 5% ($p>0.050$) was set for all statistical tests.

CHAPTER 5

RESULTS

5.1 Evaluation of feed and water consumption and feed efficiency ratio

5.1.1 Evaluation of feed consumption

The average feed values in grams (g) consumed by the animals in the different groups and the respective periods of the experiment are shown in table 5.1 and graph 5.1 The feed was offered ad *libitum.* It can be seen that the fractured group had a reduction in consumption in the 24-hour period and a progressive increase in the following periods, when compared to the malnourished fractured group. There were no measurements of feed wastage.

Table 5.1 - Average feed consumption values (in g) of the animals per group according to the sacrifice period

	Trial period				
Gru	24 hours	7 days	15 days	30 days	90 days
	a±dp	mean±SD	mean±SD	mean±SD	mean±SD
Fractured	9,4±0,0	10,2±0,0	11,0±0,0	13,9±0,0	20,1±2,0
Fractured Malnourished	17,6±3,7	16,8±4,1	18,6±0,2	19,3±1,4	19,4±2,7
Malnourished	19,5±3,3	14,5±2,3	17,4±1,3	17,8±0,0	17,7±0,0

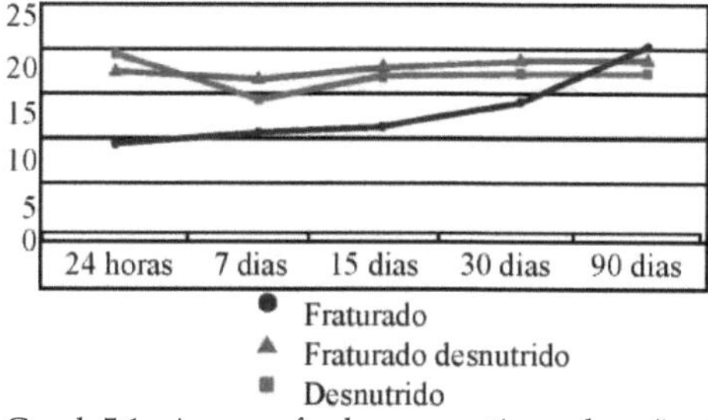

Graph 5.1 - Average feed consumption values (in g) of the animals per group according to the sacrifice period

The Analysis of Variance for feed consumption showed a significant difference between the groups for the 24-hour period (p= 0.011), the 15-day period (p <0.001) and the 30-day period (p= 0.001), with no significant difference for the 7-day period (p= 0.060) and the 90-day period (p= 0.379).

Tukey's test or Dunnett's test identified the groups that differed from each other, with FD x F groups being statistically significant at 15 days, with p= 0.001 and F x D groups, with p= 0.031; and in the 30-day period, the FD x F groups, with p= 0.048 and not being significant for the 24-hour period, the FD x F groups, with p= 0.127; FD x D groups, with p= 0.866 and F x D, with p= 0.069; in the 15-day period, the FD x D groups, with p= 0.492 and in the 30-day period, the FD x D groups, with p= 0.401 and F x D, with p > 0.999.

The Friedman test showed a significant difference between the observation periods in group F, with p= 0.017. The Student's *t-test* for paired data was then applied to identify the moments that differed from the others, and was statistically significant for the periods of 24 hours x 90 days, with p= 0.012; 7 days X 90 days, with p= 0.014; 15 days X 90 days, with p= 0.017 and 30 days X 90 days, with p= 0.035. There was no significant difference between the observation periods in the FD group, with p= 0.970 and in the D group, with p= 0.080.

5.1.2Evaluation of water consumption

The mean values for water in millilitres (ml) consumed by the animals in the different groups and the respective periods of the experiment are shown in table 5.2 and graph 5.2. Water was offered ad *libitum.* It can be seen that there was no water consumption in the fractured group between 24 hours and 7 days. There was a higher average consumption per period in the malnourished fractured group in all periods except the 7-day period, when compared to the others.

Table 5.2 Average water consumption values (in ml) of the animals per group according to the experimental period

	Trial period				
Group	**24 hours**	**7 days**	**15 days**	**30 days**	**90 days**
	a±dp	mean±SD	mean±SD	mean±SD	mean±SD
Fractured	0±0,0	45,2±0,0	50,0±0,0	40,2±0,0	56,6±0,5
Fractured Malnourishe d	65,5±7,3	50,9±25,6	60,1±0,5	52,3±18,1	63,9±2,5
Malnourishe d	53,5±12,9	58,6±7,9	53,4±5,3	50,1±0,0	44,3±0,0

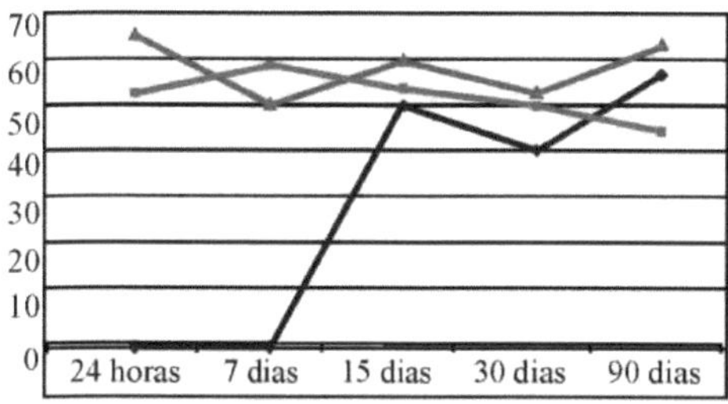

◆ Faturado
▲ Faturado desnutrido
■ Desnutrido

Graph 5.2 - Average water consumption values (ml) per group according to the experimental period

The Analysis of Variance for water consumption showed a significant difference between the groups for the 24-hour period (p< 0.001), the 15-day period (p= 0.018) and the 90-day period (p< 0.001), while it was not significant for the 7-day period (p= 0.594) and the 30-day period (p= 0.380).

Tukey's test or Dunnett's test identified the groups that differed from each other, with FD x F being statistically significant in the 24-hour period, with p= 0.009 and F x D, with p= 0.039; and in the 15-day period, FD X F, with p= 0.002; in the 90-day period, groups FD x D, with p= 0.012; and F x D, with p= 0.001 and not being significant for the 24-hour period, groups FD X D, with p= 0.507; in the 15-day period, groups FD x D, with p= 0.312; and F X D, with p= 0.665; and in the 90-day period, groups FD x F, with p= 0.073.

The Friedman test showed a significant difference between the observation periods in group F, with p= 0.017. The Student's *t-test* for paired data was then applied to identify the moments that differed from the others, and was statistically significant for the periods of 24 hours x 90 days, with p< 0.001; 7 days X 90 days, with p= 0.001; 15 days X 90 days, with p= 0.002 and 30 days x 90 days, with p< 0.001. There was no significant difference between the observation periods in the FD group, with p= 0.760 and in the D group, with p= 0.231.

5.1.2 Evaluation of the Food Efficiency Coefficient - FEC

To calculate the EAA, the relationship between weekly feed consumption and the weight of the animal per period in each group was analysed. For this purpose

the time each group consumed the feed as follows:

- For the fractured group, the 24-hour period was one day, the 7-day period was one week, the 15-day period was two weeks, the 30-day period was four weeks and the 90-day period was twelve weeks;

- For the malnourished group, the 24-hour period was four weeks and one day, the 7-day period was five weeks, the 15-day period was six weeks, the 30-day period was eight weeks and the 90-day period was sixteen weeks;

- for the malnourished fractured group, the 24-hour period was four weeks and one day, the 7-day period was five weeks, the 15-day period was six weeks, the 30-day period was eight weeks and the 90-day period was sixteen weeks.

The calculation of the coefficient of food efficiency for the groups and their respective experimental periods can be seen in table 5.3 and graph 5.3.

Table 5.3 - Mean (± standard deviation) of the food efficiency coefficient for the fractured, malnourished fractured and malnourished groups according to the experimental period

Trial period	Fractured group	Malnourished fractured group	Malnourished group
24 hours	-0,2 (±0,1)	0,4 (±0,2)	0,4 (±0,3)
7 days	0,4 (±0,3)	-1,5(±0,4)	0,3 (±0,1)
15 days	0,3 (±0,1)	-0,3 (±0,1)	0,5 (±0,3)
30 days	0,3 (±0,1)	0 (±0,2)	0,6 (±0,3)
90 days	0,9 (±0,2)	0,2 (±0,4)	1,4 (±0,4)

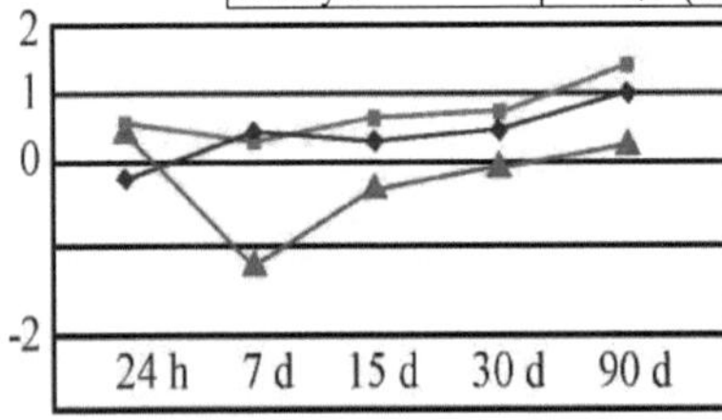

Graph 5.3 - Average values of the food efficiency coefficient for the groups according to the experimental periods

It was observed that in the fractured group, CEA remained negative at 24 hours; at 15 days, there was a drop in CEA compared to the 7-day period. In the malnourished group, a drop in CEA was observed at 7 days and in the malnourished fractured group, CEA was negative at 7 days and 15 days.

The *Analysis of Variance* for the coefficient of food efficiency showed a significant difference between the groups for the periods of 7 days, with $p < 0.001$; 15 days, with $p = 0.016$ and 90 days, with p= 0.017, and was not significant for the periods of 24 hours, with p= 0.408 and 30 days, with p= 0.056.

Tukey's test and *Dunnett's test* were used to identify the groups that differed from each other, with the FD x F group being statistically significant for the 7-day period, with p= 0.007; FD x D, with p= 0.022 and not being significant for the 7-day period, the F X D groups, with p= 0.870; for the 15-day period, the FD x F groups, with p= 0.070; FD X D, with p= 0.095; F x D, with p= 0.677 and for the 90-day period, the FD x F groups, with p= 0.168; FD x D, with p= 0.052 and F x D, with p= 0.342.

The *Friedman test* showed a significant difference between the observation periods in group F, with p= 0.043. The *Student's* t-test for paired data was then applied to identify the moments that differed from the others, and was statistically significant for the periods of 24 hours x 7 days, with p= 0.034; 24 hours x 30 days, with p= 0.009; 24 hours x 90 days, with p= 0.006; 7 days x 90 days, with p= 0.015 and 30 days x 90 days, with p= 0.042. There was no significant difference between the observation periods of 24 hours x 15 days, with p= 0.082; 7 days x 15 days, with p= 0.625; 7 days x 30 days, with p= 0.808; 15 days x 30 days, with p= 0.478 and 15 days x 90 days, with p= 0.104. There was also no significant difference between the observation periods in the FD group, with p= 0.094 and in the D group, with p= 0.126.

5.2 . Animal weight assessment

The average weight values in grams (g) of the animals and their respective groups and experimental periods are shown in Graphs 5.4, 5.5 and 5.6 and Appendix G.

The average weight of the animals showed that in the fractured group, the animals had a slight reduction in weight at 24 hours and 15 days, but no loss of weight compared to the initial period of the experiment. At 30 and 90 days there was an increase in weight (Graph 5.4).

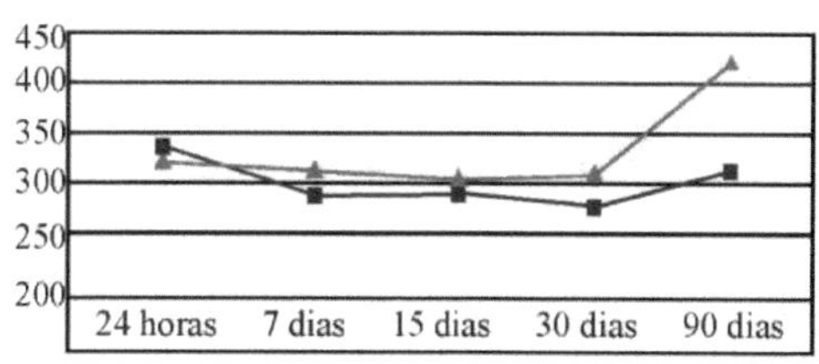

Graph 5.4 - Average weight (in g) of animals in the fractured group, submitted to condylar fracture at the time of the fracture and at sacrifice, according to the experimental periods

In the animals in the malnourished fractured group, it was observed that on the day of the fracture, all had an increase in weight compared to the beginning of the experiment, but in the 7 and 15 day periods, they lost weight, recovering it in the 30 and 90 day periods.

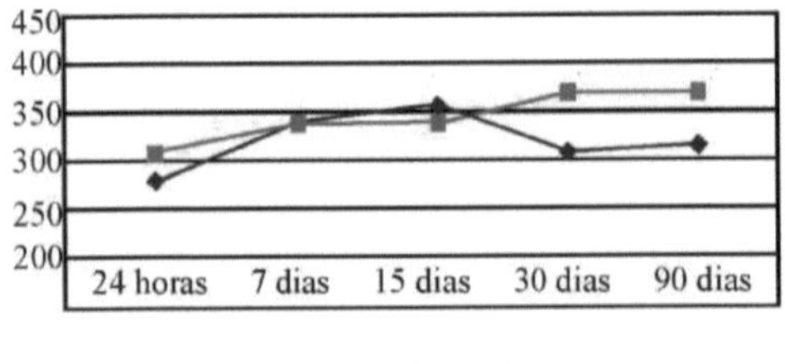

Graph 5.5 - Average weight (in g) of animals in the malnourished fracture group, subjected to malnutrition and condylar fracture at the start of the study and at sacrifice, according to experimental periods

The animals in the malnourished group had an increase in weight in all periods.

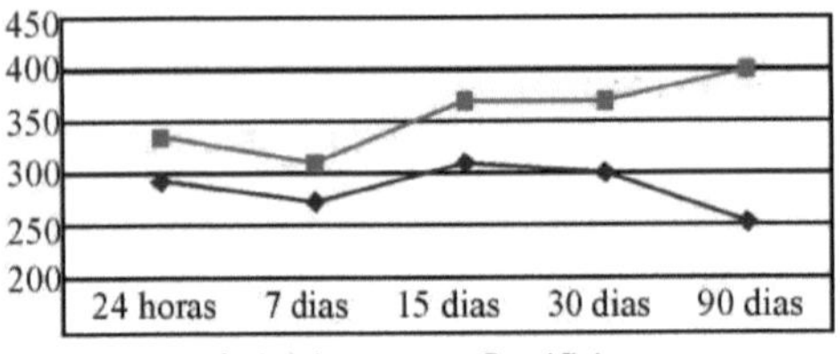

Graph 5.6 - Average weight (in g) of the animals in the malnourished group submitted to malnutrition without condylar fracture at the start of the study and at sacrifice, according to the experimental periods

Analysis of Variance was used to assess the weight of the animals and found a significant difference between the groups for the 24-hour period (p= 0.047), the 15-day period (p= 0.023) and the 90-day period (p= 0.037), while it was not significant for the 7-day period (p= 0.213) and the 30-day period (p= 0.277).

Tukey's test or *Dunnett's test* identified the groups that differed from each other, with FD x F being statistically significant for the 15-day period, with p= 0.044, and FD X F not being significant for the 24-hour period, with p= 0.176; FD x D, with p= 0.958; F x D, with p= 0.148; for the 15-day period, the FD x D groups, with p= 0.135; F X D, with p= 0.506, and for the 90-day period, the FD x F groups, with p= 0.137; FD x D, with p= 0.096 and F x D, with p= 0.663.

The *Friedman test* showed a significant difference between the observation periods in group F, with p= 0.043. The *Student*'s "t" test for paired data was then applied to identify the moments that differed from the others, and was statistically significant for the periods of 24 hours x 15 days, with p= 0.041; 24 hours X 90 days, with p= 0.012; 7 days X 90 days, with p= 0.005; 15 days x 90 days, with p= 0.044. There was no significant difference between the observation periods of 24 hours x 7 days, with p= 0.052; 24 hours x 30 days, with p= 0.068; 7 days x 15 days, with p= 0.899; 7 days x 30 days, with p= 0.884; 15 days x 30 days, with p= 0.294 and 30 days x 90 days, with p= 0.066. There was also no significant difference between the observation periods in the FD group, with p= 0.113 and in the D group, with p= 0.092.

5.3 Biochemical blood tests

The average values of the biochemical blood tests for total proteins, albumin, calcium, alkaline phosphatase, serum iron and creatinine for the different groups according to the experimental periods are shown in table 5.4. It can be seen that the malnourished fractured group had lower total protein and calcium values in all periods, as well as albumin in the initial periods, with total protein values recovering later on. As for alkaline phosphatase values, the malnourished fractured group showed a predominance in the initial periods, returning to values similar to the other groups later on. For serum iron values, the malnourished group showed a predominance from 7 days to 30 days, returning to values similar to the other groups later on. Creatinine values fluctuated between the three groups for the experimental periods. The values for each biochemical test for the various groups according to the experimental period are presented below in graph form, along with the corresponding statistical analyses. The negative control and reference values are shown in Appendix H.

Table 5.4 - Average values of the biochemical blood tests of the animals per group in each experimental period.

	Groups		
Sacrifice period/tests	**Fractured**	**Fractured malnourished**	**Malnourished**
24 hours	Mean ± SD	Mean ± SD	Mean ± SD
Total protein (g/dL)	8,4 ± 2,0	5,1 ± 0,7	5,2 ± 0,8
Albumin (g/dL)	3,1 ± 0,7	5,1 ± 0,7	1,9 ± 0,5
Serum calcium (mg/dL)	8,6 ± 1,9	5,6 ± 0,2	9,4 ± 0,7
Alkaline phosphatase (U/L)	23,8 ± 3,0	42,9 ± 25,5	31,5 ± 10,4
Serum iron (ug/ dL)	205,0 ± 38,2	289,9 ± 46,7	253,4 ± 42,9
Creatinine K(mg/ dL)	0,5 ± 0,7	0,4 ± 0,8	1,5 ± 1,2
7 days			
Total protein (g/dL)	9,1 ± 2,2	4,4 ± 0,9	5,9 ± 1,3
Albumin (g/dL)	2,7 ± 0,9	1,9 ± 0,7	2,0 ± 0,4
Serum calcium (mg/dL)	9,9 ± 0,9	5,6 ± 0,4	10,1 ± 0,4
Alkaline phosphatase (U/L)	38,6 ± 5,9	59,2 ± 27,4	37,0 ± 2,1
Serum iron (ug/ dL)	178,5 ± 41,1	242,1 ± 67,4	466,0 ± 27,5
Creatinine K(mg/ dL)	0,2 ± 0,9	1,7 ± 2,0	1,1 ± 1,0

15 days			
Total protein (g/dL)	8,8 ± 4,6	4,9 ± 1,0	5,2 ± 0,1
Albumin (g/dL)	1,8 ± 0,6	1,9 ± 0,6	2,0 ± 0,2
Serum calcium (mg/ dL)	9,6 ± 0,7	6,1 ± 0,1	9,1 ± 1,3
Alkaline phosphatase (U/L)	29,4 ± 3,6	37,3 ± 2,5	54 ± 6,1
Serum iron (ug/ dL)	199,3 ± 42,5	197,3 ± 49,3	233,0 ± 54,4
Creatinine K(mg/ dL)	0,4 ± 0,2	0,3 ± 0,2	1,8 ± 1,6
30 days			
Total protein (g/dL)	8,9 ± 2,1	3,9 ± 0,7	7,3 ± 1,2
Albumin (g/dL)	2,8 ± 0,1	1,7 ± 0,2	2,3 ± 0,9
Serum calcium (mg/ dL)	10,0 ± 0,5	6,0 ± 0,1	9,3 ± 1,4
Alkaline phosphatase (U/L)	48,2 ± 11,7	19,2 ± 6,6	39,2 ± 14,9
Serum iron (ug/ dL)	249,8 ± 48,9	269,2 ± 79,0	311,6 ± 35,9
Creatinine K(mg/ dL)	1,0 ± 1,5	0,4 ± 0,3	0,6 ± 0,2
90 days			
Total protein (g/dL)	8,0 ± 0,8	5,9 ± 1,7	6,3 ± 0,7
Albumin (g/dL)	2,4 ± 0,1	3,1 ± 1,1	2,1 ± 0,4
Serum calcium (mg/ dL)	10,3 ± 0,7	6,8 ± 0,2	10,1 ± 0,0
Alkaline phosphatase (U/L)	37,1 ± 7,4	38,0 ± 7,9	37,7 ± 7,5
Serum iron (ug/ dL)	281,7 ± 51,7	281,3 ± 124,8	233,4 ± 11,5
Creatinine K(mg/ dL)	0,3 ± 0,2	0,1 ± 0,1	0,5 ± 0,1

The total protein values of the animals in the fractured group did not change significantly in all periods. The animals in the malnourished and undernourished fractured group had lower values in all periods when compared to the fractured group. The animals in the malnourished fractured group had a decrease in total protein over the 30-day period and the malnourished group had an increase when compared to the others (Graph 5.7).

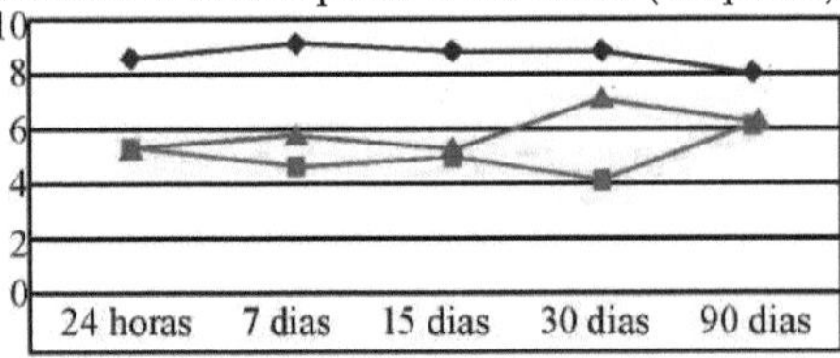

Graph 5. 7 - Average total protein values (g/dL) of the animals per group in each experimental period

The analysis of variance for the mean total protein values showed a significant difference between the groups for the 24-hour period (p = 0.036), the 7-day period (p = 0.028) and the 30-day period (p = 0.015), while the 15-day period (p = 0.238) and the 90-day period (p = 0.123) were not significant.

Tukey's test or Dunnett's test were used to identify the groups that differed from each other, with no significant difference in the 24-hour period: the FD x F group, with p = 0.193; the FD x D group, with p = 0.999; and the F x D group, with p = 0.201; FD x D, with p= 0.999 and F x D, with p= 0.201, in the 7-day period, the FD x F groups, with p= 0.110; FD x D, with p= 0.424 and F x D, with p= 0.251 and in the 30-day period, the FD x F groups, with p= 0.099; FD X D, with p= 0.055 and F x D, with p= 0.635.

When the Friedman test was applied, there was no significant difference between the FD group (p= 0.189), the F group (p = 0.976) and the D group (p= 0.483).

Albumin values were lower in the malnourished fractured group between 24 hours and 30 days, in the malnourished group between 24 hours and 15 days and in the fractured group after 15 days. In the malnourished fractured group, there was an increase in the 90-day period when compared to the others (Graph 5.8).

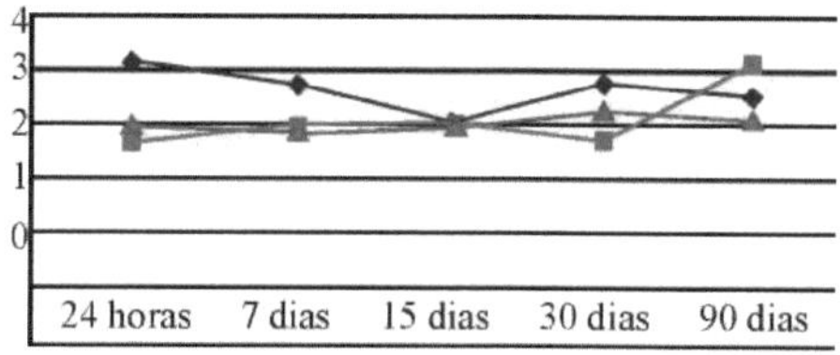

Graph 5.8 - Average albumin values (g/dL) of the animals per group in each experimental period

The Analysis of Variance for the mean albumin values showed a significant difference between the groups for the 24-hour period, with p= 0.043, and was not significant for the 7-day period, with p= 0.393, the 15-day period, with p= 0.952, the 30-day period, with p= 0.125 and the 90-day period, with p = 0.258.

Tukey's test or Dunnett's test identified the groups that differed from each other, with no significant difference in the 24-hour period: FD x F, with p = 0.121; FD x D, with p = 0.923 and F x

D, with p = 0.194.

When the Friedman test was applied, there was no significant difference between the FD group (p= 0.155), the F group (p = 0.074) and the D group (p= 0.987).

As for serum calcium values, there was a reduction in all periods in the malnourished fractured group when compared to the others. The fractured and malnourished groups had similar rates, despite a slight increase in the 7-day period, and remained equivalent until the end (Graph 5.9).

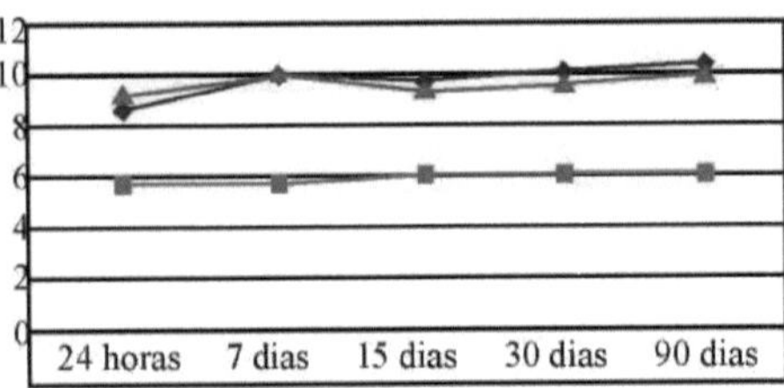

◆ Fraturado
■ Fraturado Desnutrido
▲ Desnutrido

Graph 5.9 - Mean serum calcium values (mg/dL) of the animals per group in each experimental period

The Analysis of Variance for the mean calcium values showed a significant difference between the groups for the 24-hour period (p= 0.015), the 7-day period (p= 0.001), the 15-day period (p= 0.004), the 30-day period (p= 0.003) and the 90-day period (p< 0.001).

Tukey's test or Dunnett's test identified the groups that differed from each other, with FD x D being statistically significant in the 24-hour period, with p= 0.011; for the 7-day period, FD x F, with p= 0.017 and FD x D, with p= 0.007; for the 15-day period, FD x F, with p= 0.022; for the 30-day period, the FD x F groups, with p= 0.011 and for the 90-day period, the FD x F groups, with p= 0.012 and FD x D, with p= 0.002, with no significance in the 24-hour period for the FD X F groups, with p= 0.219 and F x D, with p= 0.844; for the 7-day period, groups F x D, with p= 0.976; for the 15-day period, groups FD x D, with p= 0.107, F x D, with p= 0.904; for the 30-day period, groups FD x D, with p= 0.120 and F x D, with p= 0.820 and for the 90-day period, groups F x D, with p= 0.974.

When the Friedman test was applied, there was no significant difference between the FD group (p = 0.189), the F group (p = 0.505) and the D group (p = 0.308).

For the alkaline phosphatase values, the malnourished fractured group showed a predominance at the beginning and an increase in the 7-day period, followed by a reduction with lower values at 30 days when compared to the others, with an increase at 90 days, returning to values similar to the other groups. The malnourished group also showed a reduction at 30 days and was similar to the others at 90 days (Graph 5.10).

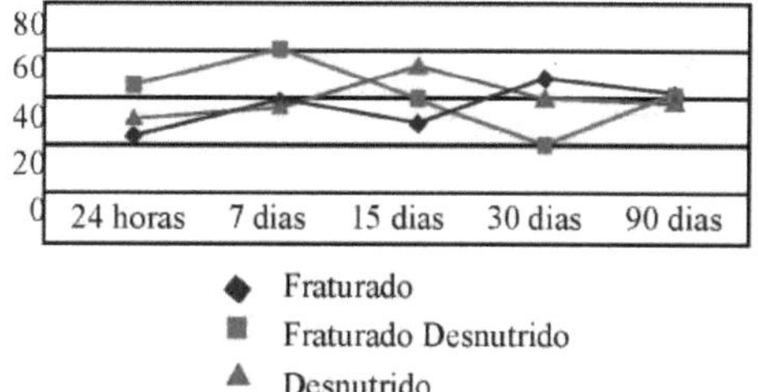

Graph 5.10 - Average alkaline phosphatase values (U/L) of the animals per group in each experimental period

The analysis of variance for the mean alkaline phosphatase values showed a significant difference between the groups for the 15-day period, with p= 0.003, and was not significant for the 24-hour period, with p= 0.411; the 7-day period, with p= 0.340; the 30-day period, with p= 0.055 and the 90-day period, with p= 0.988.

Tukey's test or Dunnett's test were used to identify the groups that differed from each other, with no significant difference in the 15-day period, the FD x F groups, with p= 0.099; FD x D, with p= 0.230 and F x D, with p= 0.120.

The Friedman test showed a significant difference between the observation periods in the FD group, with p= 0.043. The Student's *t-test* for paired data was then applied to identify the moments that differed from the others, and was statistically significant for the periods of 15 d x 30 d, with p= 0.017 and 30d x 90d, with p= 0.035. There was no significant difference between the observation periods of 24 hours x 7 days, with p= 0.082; 24 hours x 15 days, with p= 0.769; 24 hours x

30 d, with p= 0.223; 24 hs x 90d, with p= 0.724; 7d x 15d, with p= 0.283; 7 d x 30d, with p= 0.093; 7d x 90d, with p= 0.203 and 15d x 90d, with p= 0.887. There was no significant difference for groups F, with p = 0.092 and group D, with p= 0.406.

Mean serum iron levels fell in the malnourished fractured group over the 15-day period, with values recovering after 90 days. The fractured group had the lowest values compared to the others. The malnourished group had an increase at 7 days, with a drop immediately after 15 days (Graph 5.11).

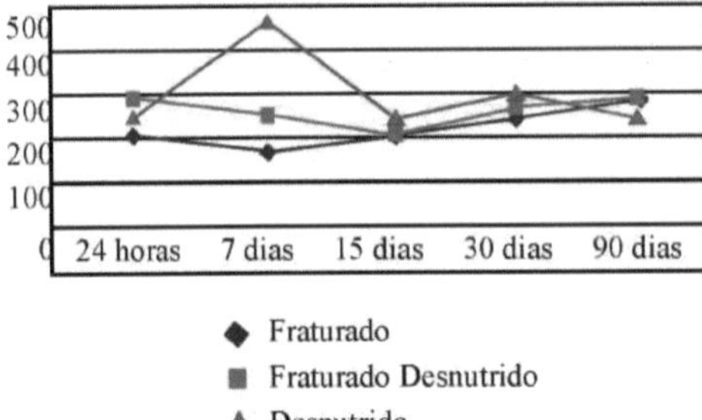

Graph 5.11 - Mean serum iron values (ug/ dL) of the animals per group in each experimental period

The Analysis of Variance for the mean serum iron values showed a significant difference between the groups for the 7-day period, with p= 0.004, and was not significant for the 24-hour period, with p= 0.126; the 15-day period, with p= 0.692; the 30-day period, with p= 0.572 and the 90-day period, with p= 0.797.

Tukey's test and Dunnett's test were used to identify the groups that differed from each other: there was a significant difference in the 7-day period between groups FD x D, with p= 0.040 and F x D, with p= 0.007, and there was no significant difference in the 7-day period between groups FD x F, with p= 0.508.

When the Friedman test was applied, there was no significant difference between the FD group (p = 0.189), the F group (p = 0.102) and the D group (p = 0.199).

For creatinine values, in the malnourished fractured group, there was a rise in the 7-day period and an equal fall in the 15-day period. In the other groups, the peak was between 15 days (malnourished group) and 30 days (fractured group) (Graph 5.12).

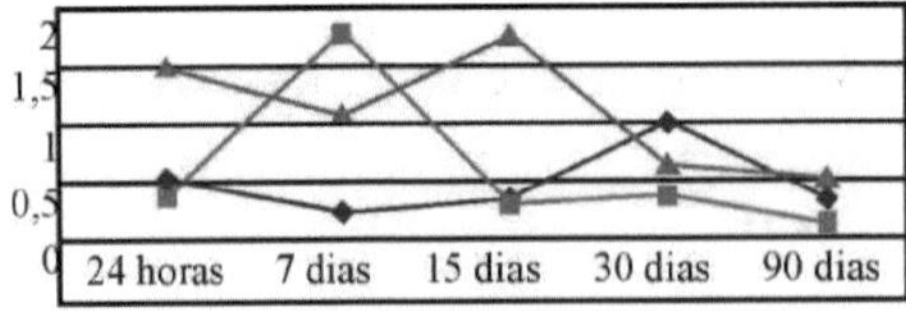

Graph 5.12 - Average creatinine values (mg/dL) of the animals per group in each period

The Analysis of Variance for the mean creatinine values showed a significant difference between the groups for the 90-day period, with p= 0.037, and was not significant for the 24-hour period, with p= 0.166; the 7-day period, with p= 0.314; the 15-day period, with p= 0.181 and the 30-day period, with p= 0.737.

Tukey's test and Dunnett's test were used to identify the groups that differed from each other, with no significant difference over the 90-day period: the FD x F groups, with p= 0.394; the FD x D groups, with p= 0.066 and the F x D groups, with p= 0.414.

When the Friedman test was applied, there was no significant difference between the FD group (p = 0.707), the F group (p = 0.344) and the D group (p = 0.525).

5.4 Haematological tests

5.4.1 Leucogram

The percentage distribution of leucocytes in the individual count of the negative control, the reference values (MITRUKA; RAWNSLEY, 1977) and adaptation of Sanderson and Philips (1981), and the values of the total and individual leucocyte counts are shown in Appendix J.

The average global leucocyte count values for the different groups according to the experimental periods can be seen in graph 5.13. The leucocyte count in the malnourished fractured group was slightly higher than normal at 24 hours. At 7 days, the values also increased, especially in the malnourished fractured and malnourished groups, while the fractured group had a reduction in the overall leucocyte count during this period. At 15 days, all groups showed a reduction in the number of leucocytes close to the limit values. At 30 days, the malnourished fractured group showed high leucocyte values, while the other groups had normal values during this period. By 90 days, the global leucocyte count values had practically equalised, reaching normal limits. When analysing the overall leukocyte count, it can be seen that at 15 days there was only one statistically significant difference. However, when the three groups were crossed, there was no significant difference (Graph 5.13).

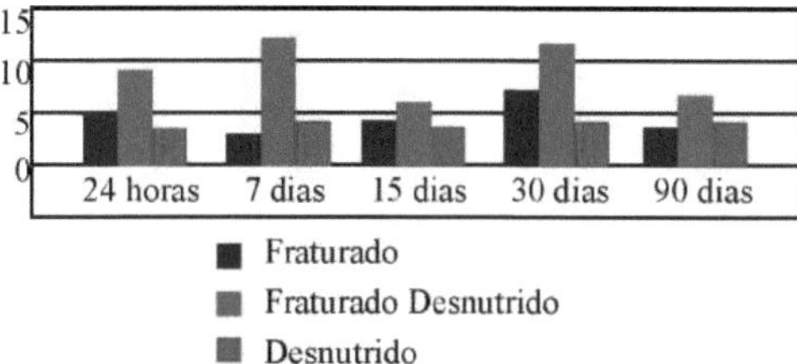

Graph 5.13 - Average global leucocyte count (W/mm³) of the animals in the different groups

according to the experimental periods

Analysis of Variance for the total leucocyte count showed a significant difference between the groups for the 15-day period, with p= 0.039, and was not significant for the 24-hour periods, with p= 0.069; 7 days, with p= 0.081; 30 days, with p= 0.485 and 90 days, with p= 0.439.

Using the Tukey test or Dunnett's test, there was no significant difference between groups over the 15-day period for the FD x F groups, with p= 0.360; the FD x D groups, with p= 0.087 and the F x D groups, with p= 0.346.

When the Friedman test was applied, there was no significant difference between the FD group (p = 0.155), the F group (p = 0.549) and the D group (p = 0.218).

The average values for the individual percentage of lymphocytes, monocytes and neurophils in the different groups according to the experimental periods are shown in graphs 5.14, 5.15 and 5.16. In terms of lymphocytes, group F had an increase at 30 and 90 days, group FD had an increase at 30 and 90 days and group D had an increase at 24 hours and 7 days. Monocytes increased in the F group at 24 hours and 7 days, in the FD group at 24 hours and 30 days and in the D group at 15 and 30 days. In neutrophils, group F had an increase in 15 days, group FD had an increase in 24 hours, 7 and 15 days and group D had no changes in all the experimental periods.

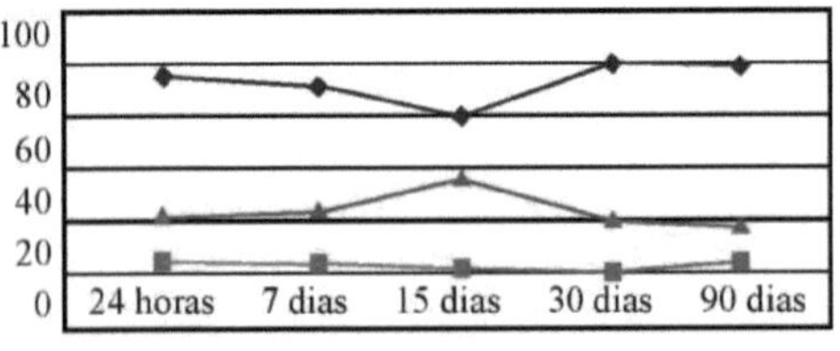

Graph 5.14 - Individual percentage values of lymphocytes, monocytes and neutrophils in the fractured group according to the experimental periods

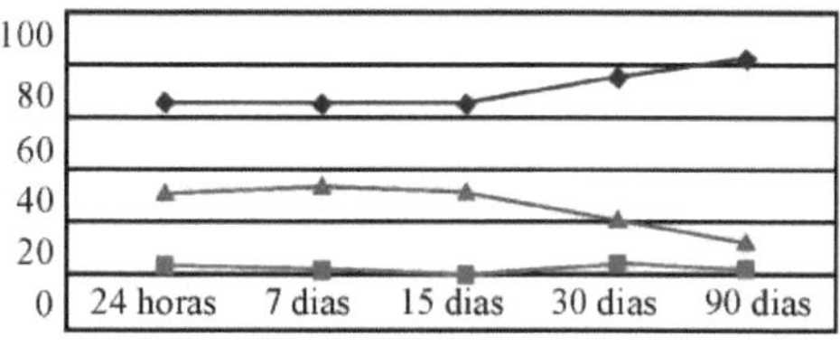

Graph 5.15 - Individual percentage values of lymphocytes, monocytes and neutrophils in the malnourished fractured group according to the experimental periods

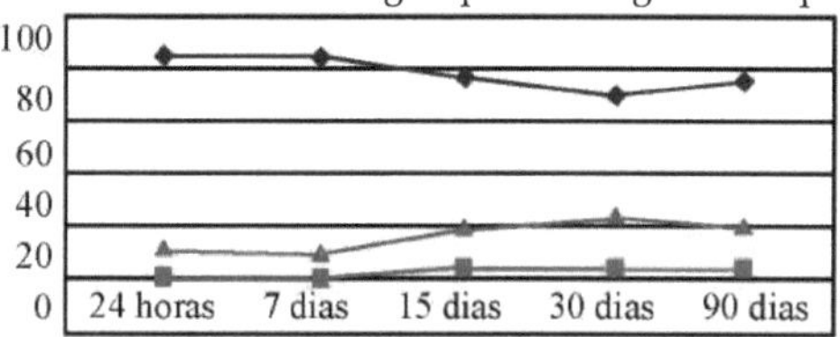

Graph 5.16 - Individual percentage values of lymphocytes, monocytes and neutrophils in the malnourished group according to the experimental periods

The Analysis of Variance showed a significant difference between the groups for the lymphocyte values at 24 hours (p< 0.001), 7 days (p= 0.019), 30 days (p= 0.043) and 15 days (p= 0.203) and 90 days (p= 0.439). The

Tukey or *Dunnett's test* identified the groups that differed from each other, with a significant difference in the 24-hour period for the FD x D group with p= 0.019 and the F x D group with p= 0.002; for the 7-day period, for the F x D groups, with p= 0.038 and for the 30-day period, with p= 0.010 and there was no significant difference in the 24-hour period, in the FD x F groups, with p= 0.246; in the 7-day period, in the FD x F groups, with p= 0.655 and FD x D, with p= 0.100 and in the 30-day period, the FD x F groups, with p= 0.706 and FD x D groups, with p= 0.424. The *Friedman test* showed a significant difference for group F, with p= 0.023. The *Student's* t-test for paired data was then applied to identify the moments that differed from the others, and was statistically significant for the periods of 24 hours x 30 days, with p= 0.003 and 24 hours x 90 days, with p= 0.009. There was no significant difference between the observation periods of 24h x 7d, with p= 0.549; 24h x 15d, with p= 0.187; 7d x 15d, with p= 0.190, 7d x 30d, with p= 0.074; 7d x 90d, with p= 0.099; 15d x 30d, with p= 0.111; 15d x 90d, with p= 0.122 and 30d x 90d, with p= 0.423. And for group D, with p= 0.033, we also applied the *Student's t-test* for paired data, identifying the moments that differed from the others, being statistically significant for the periods of 24 hours x 30 days, with p= 0.010; 24 hours x 90 days, with p= 0.015; 7 days x 15 days, with p= 0.011; 7 days x 30 days, with p= 0.015; 15 days x 30 days, with p= 0.023. There was no significant difference between the observation periods of 24h x 7d, with p= 0.785; 24h x 15d, with p= 0.057; 7d x 90d, with p= 0.179; 15d x 90d, with p= 0.930 and 30d x 90d, with p= 0.184. There was no significant difference for the FD groups, with p = 0.053.

The *Analysis of Variance* showed no significant difference between the groups for the 24-hour periods, with p= 0.221; for 7 days, with p= 0.572; for 15 days, with p= 0.272; for 30 days, with p= 0.437 and for 90 days, with p= 0.282. When the *Friedman test was* applied, there was no significant difference for group FD with p= 0.809, for group F with p= 0.230 and for group D with p= 0.155.

The *Analysis of Variance* showed a significant difference between the groups for the 24-hour period, with p= 0.002; for 7 days, with p= 0.013 and was not significant for the 15-day period, with p= 0.305; for 30 days, with p= 0.481 and for 90 days, with p= 0.865. Tukey's test or Dunnett's test identified the groups that differed from each other, with a significant difference in the 24-hour period between groups FD x D, with p= 0.045 and F x D, with p= 0.004; in the 7-day period, groups F x D, with p= 0.026 and there was no significant difference in the 24-hour period for groups FD x F, with p= 0.246 and for the 7-day period, groups FD x F, with p= 0.532 and FD x D, with p= 0.094. The Friedman test showed a significant difference for group D, with p= 0.041. The Student's t-test for paired data was then applied to identify the moments that differed from the others, with a statistically significant difference for the 24h x 30d periods, with p= 0.038; 24h x 90d, with p= 0.009 and 7d x 15d, with p= 0.044; there was no significant difference between the 24h x 7d periods, with p= 0.910; 24h x 15d, p= 0.130; 7d x 30d, p= 0.095; 7d x 90d, p= 0.185; 15d x 30d, p= 0.401; 15d x 90d, p= 0.853 and 30d x 90d, p= 0.122. There was no significant difference for the FD group, with p= 0.092 and the F group, with p= 0.169.

The average values for the individual percentage of rods, basophils and eosinophils in the different groups according to the experimental periods are shown in graphs 5.17, 5.18 and 5.19.

The malnourished fractured group showed an increase in rods within 24 hours, and the malnourished group an increase in rods within 7 days.

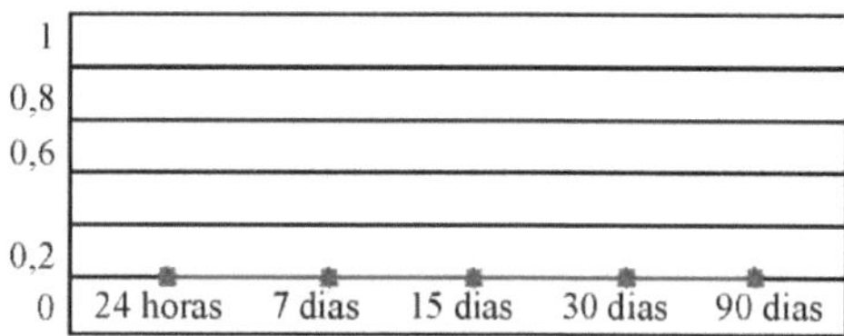

▲ Bastonetes
■ Basófilos
◆ Eosinófilos

Graph 5.17 - Individual percentage of rods, basophils and eosinophils in the fractured group according to the experimental periods

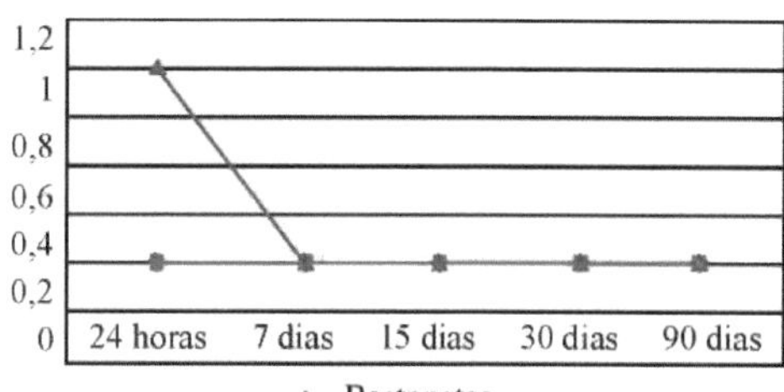

▲ Bastonetes
■ Basófilos
◆ Eosinófilos

Graph 5.18 - Individual percentage values of rods, basophils and eosinophils in the malnourished fractured group according to the experimental periods

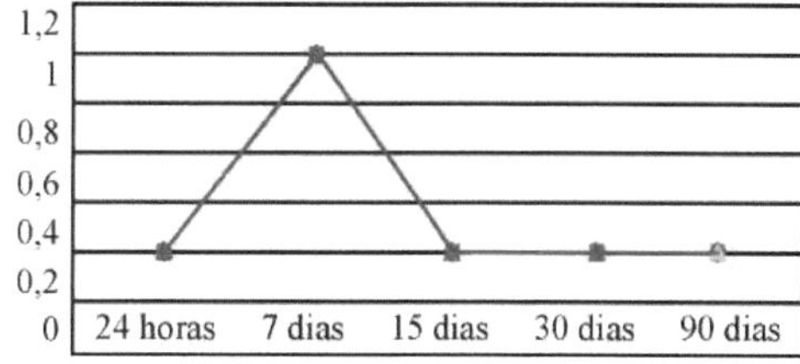

▲ Bastonetes
■ Basófilos
◆ Eosinófilos

Graph 5.19 - Individual percentage of rods, basophils and eosinophils in the malnourished group according to the experimental periods

The Analysis of Variance showed no significant differences in the values of the rods for all periods, 24 hours, 7 days, 15 days, 30 days and 90 days, with $p > 0.999$. Tukey's test and Dunnett's test did not identify any groups that differed from one another. When the Friedman test was applied, there was a significant difference for the FD group, with $p = 0.017$. The *Student's t-test* for paired data was then applied, and the 24-hour time point was identified, which differed from the others and there was no significant difference for the F and D groups, with p > 0.999.

Analysis of Variance found no significant differences in basophil values for all periods: 24 hours, 7 days, 15 days, 30 days and 90 days, with p > 0.999. Tukey's test and Dunnett's test did not identify any groups that differed from one another. When the Friedman test was applied, there were no significant differences between groups F, FD and D, with p > 0.999 for all groups.

The analysis of variance showed no significant differences in the eosinophil values for all periods: 24 hours, 7 days, 15 days, 30 days and 90 days, with p > 0.999. Tukey's test and Dunnett's test did not identify any groups that differed from one another. When the Friedman test was applied, there was a significant difference for group D, with p= 0.017, and then the *Student's t-test* for paired data was applied, identifying the 7-day point, which differed from the others and there was no significant difference for groups F and FD , with p > 0.999.

5.5 Cephalometric measurements using radiographs

The "A" angle was measured in the axial view to quantify the deviation between the mandibular midline and the maxillary midline. The values obtained when measuring angle A by group, according to the period of sacrifice, are shown in Table 5.5. There was an increase in the deviation at 15 days for the fractured and malnourished fractured groups and a greater deviation at 90 days for the malnourished fractured group, when compared to the others.

Table 5.5 - Measurements of the "A" angle obtained in the axial view of the skull, according to group and sacrifice period. Values in degrees

	Measurements		
	Groups		
Sacrifice periods	Fractured Mean ± sd	Fractured malnourished Mean ± sd	Malnourished Mean± SD
24 hours	0,7±0,4	0,4±0,1	0,5±0,3
7 days	O,4±0,1	1,1±0,5	0,1±0,0
15 days	1,8±0,7	2,9±3,4	0,2±0,0
30 days	0,5±0,1	0,8±0,3	0,3±0,1
90 days	0,5±0,0	6,8±0,3	0,4±0,0

Analysis of Variance for measurements of the "A" angle in the axial view of the skull revealed a significant difference between the groups at 7 days, with p= 0.014; at 30 days, with p= 0.038 and at 90 days, with p< 0.001, while it was not significant at 24 hours, with p= 0.494 and 15 days, with p= 0.336. *Tukey's test* or *Dunnett's test* identified the groups that differed from each other, with a significant difference in the 90-day period for the FD x F groups with p= 0.002 and FD x D, with p=

0.001; and there was no significant difference in the 7-day period for groups FD x F, with p= 0.244, FD x D, with p = 0.145 and F X D, with p= 0.055; in the 30-day period for groups FD x F, with p= 0.415, FD x D, with p= 0.163 and F x D, with p= 0.199 and in the 90-day period for groups F x D, with p= 0.279. When the *Friedman test* was applied, there was a significant difference for the FD group, with p= 0.043. The *Student*'s t-test for paired data was then applied and the moments that differed from the others were identified, being statistically significant for the periods of 24 hours x 90 days, with p= 0.001; 7 days X 90 days, with p= 0.006 and 30 days X 90 days, with p< 0.001. There was no significant difference between the observation periods of 24 hours x 7 days, with p= 0.104; 24 hours x 15 days, with p= 0.319; 24 hours x 30 days, with p= 0.191; 7 days x 15 days, with p= 0.423; 7 days x 30 days, with p= 0.603; 15 days x 30 days, with p= 0.407 and 15 days x 90 days, with p= 0.184 and for group D, with p= 0.048, *Student's t-test* for paired data was then applied to identify the moments that differed from the others, being statistically significant for the periods of 7 days x 30 days, with p= 0.023; 7 days X 90 days, with p= 0.002 and 30 days X 90 days, with p= 0.014. There was no significant difference between the observation periods of 24 hours x 7 days, with p= 0.102; 24 hours x 15 days, with p= 0.292; 24 hours x 30 days, with p= 0.272; 24 hours x 90 days, with p= 0.626; 7 days x 15 days, with p= 0.069; 15 days x 30 days, with p= 0.444 and 15 days x 90 days, with p= 0.057. There was no significant difference for group F, with p = 0.066.

The mean values of the measurements obtained in the maxilla, by group and side, according to the period of sacrifice, are shown in Table 5.6. For the BT-FI measurement, there was a difference in the length of the right side compared to the left at 90 days for the malnourished fractured group. For the FI-PI measurement, there was a difference in the length of the right side compared to the left for the malnourished fractured group at 15 days and 90 days.

Table 5.6 - Measurements of the maxilla obtained in the axial view of the skull, according to group and side during the sacrifice period. Values in millimetres

		Measurements			
		BT-FI		FI- PI	
Sacrifice periods	Group	LD Mean± 1 SD	LE Mean± 1 SD	LD Mean± 1 SD	LE *M* Mean ± sd
24 hours	F	22,810,7	22,910,9	8,410,5	8,9±0,4
	FD	22,511,0	22,110,8	9,0±0,4	9,3±0,8
	D	22,011,3	21,611,2	9,1±0,3	8,9±0,3
7 days	F	22,510,1	23,110,8	8,8±0,7	9,0±0,2
	FD	23,210,7	23,511,3	9,2±0,3	9,0±1,0

	D	21,910,5	22,010,3	8,9±0,1	9,3±0,3
15 days	F	22,810,3	22,510,4	8,4±0,6	8,2±1,1
	FD	23,210,6	23,010,8	9,1±1,2	10,1±1,0
	D	23,611,1	23,411,3	8,9±0,4	9,1±0,5
30 days	F	22,810,6	22,710,6	9,1±0,1	8,9±0,2
	FD	23,410,1	23,410,2	9,1±0,2	9,8±0,4
	D	23,110,8	23,110,6	9,0±0,0	9,1±0,1
90 days	F	23,910,5	23,410,5	9,6±1,1	10,311,2
	FD	24,610,3	25,810,1	11,3±0,3	10,510,6
	D	23,510,8	23,710,7	9,4±0,3	9,4±0,4

BT = tympanic bulla, FI = infra-orbital foramen, PI = incisal point, SD = standard deviation; F = fractured group, FD = malnourished fractured group, D = malnourished group; LD = right side, LE = left side.

For the BT-FI measure, the Analysis of Variance showed a significant difference between the groups, for the 90-day period, LE with p= 0.003 and not significant for the 24-hour periods, LD with p= 0.674 and LE with p= 0.354; for 7 days, LD with p= 0.076 and LE with p= 0.188; for 15 days, LD with p= 0.443 and LE with p= 0.576; for 30 days, LD with p= 0.462 and LE with p= 0.253 and for 90 days, LD with p= 0.128. Tukey's test and Dunnett's test were used to identify

the groups that differed from each other, with a significant difference in the 90-day period, LE, for the FD x F groups with p= 0.030 and there was no significant difference for the FD x D groups, with p= 0.073 and F x D, with p = 0.919. When the Friedman test was applied, there was no significant difference for groups FD, LD, with p = 0.102 and LE, with p = 0.113, group F, LD, with p = 0.144 and LE, with p = 0.444 and group D, LD, with p = 0.189 and LE, with p = 0.231. By applying the *Student's t-test* for paired data to check for possible differences between the sides, there was a statistically significant difference for the FD group in the 90-day period LD vs LE, with p= 0.029 and there was no significant difference for the 24-hour periods, LD vs LE, with p= 0.361; 7 days, LD x LE, with p= 0.458; 15 days, LD x LE, with p= 0.624 and 30 days, LD x LE, with p= 0.927; for group F, there was no significant difference for the 24-hour periods, LD x LE, with p= 0.607; 7 days, LD x LE, with p= 0.382, 15 days, LD x LE, with p= 0.077; 30 days, LD x LE, with p= 0.126 and 90 days, LD x LE, with p= 0.498. And for group D, there was also no significant difference for the periods of 24 hours, LD x LE, with p= 0425; 7 days, LD x LE, with p= 0.782; 15 days, LD x LE, with p= 0.625; 30 days, LD x LE, with p= 0.951 and 90 days, LD x LE, with p= 0.460.

For the FI-PI measure, the Analysis of Variance showed a significant difference between the groups, for the 90-day period, LD with p= 0.030 and for the 30-day period, LE with p= 0.021 and not significant for the 24-hour periods, LD with p= 0.154 and LE with p= 0.699; for 7 days, LD, with p= 0.641 and LE, with p= 0.795; for 15 days, LD, with p= 0.508 and LE, with p= 0.110; for 30 days, LD, with p= 0.446 and for 90 days, LE, with p= 0.204. Tukey's test and Dunnett's test were used to identify the groups that differed from each other, with a significant difference at 90 days, LD, for the FD x D groups with p= 0,006 and there was no significant difference for the FD x F groups with p= 0.237 and F x D with p = 0.976 and in the 30-day period, LE, there was no significant difference in the FD x F groups with p= 0.106, FD x D with p= 0.218 and F x D with p= 0.451. When the Friedman test was applied, there was no significant difference in the FD, LD group with p = 0.155 and LE group with p = 0.281, the F, LD group with p = 0.229 and LE group with p = 0.525 and the D, LD group with p = 0.229 and LE group with p = 0.189. When applying the *Student's t-test* for paired data to check for possible differences between the sides, there was a statistically significant difference for the FD group in the 15-day LD x LE period, with p= 0.016 and there was no significant difference for the 24-hour LD x LE periods, with p= 0.460; 7 days LD x LE, with p= 0.771; 30 days, LD x LE, with p= 0.123 and 90 days, LD x LE, with p= 0.056; for group F, there was a statistically significant difference in the 90-day period, LD x LE, with p= 0.005 and there was no significant difference for the 24-hour periods, LD x LE, with p= 0.227; 7 days, LD x LE, with p= 0.693, 15 days, LD x LE, with p= 0.712 and 30 days, LD x LE, with p= 0.267. For group D, there was no significant difference for the periods of 24 hours, LD x LE, with p= 0.579; 7 days, LD x LE, with p= 0.180; 15 days, LD x LE, with p= 0.511; 30 days, LD x LE, with p= 0.229 and 90 days, LD x LE, with p= 0.875.

The mean values of the mandible measurements obtained by group and side, according to the sacrifice period, are shown in Table 5.7. For the PA-II measurement, there was a difference in the length of the right side compared to the left at 15 days and 90 days for the malnourished fractured group. For the PA-PI' measurement, there was a difference in the length of the right side compared to the left for the malnourished fractured group at 30 days and the malnourished group at 90 days.

Table 5.7 - Measurements of the mandible obtained in the axial view of the skull, according to group and side and sacrifice period. Values in millimetres

		Measurements			
		PA-II		PA - PI'	
Sacrifice periods	Group	LD Average 1 dp	LE Average 1 dp	LD Average 1 dp	LE Mean ± SD
24 hours	F	10,510,4	10,810,2	22,710,6	23,1±0,4
	FD	11,010,5	11,010,6	23,611,1	23,7±1,2

	D	10,910,6	10,210,9	23,010,5	22,9±0,4
7 days	F	10,511,0	11,210,3	22,710,5	23,4±0,5
	FD	10,910,1	10,910,4	23,710,6	23,6±0,9
	D	10,510,3	11,010,5	23,010,2	23,2±0,2
15 days	F	10,910,4	10,910,2	22,910,2	23,4±1,1
	FD	10,210,4	10,810,4	23,410,3	23,6±0,7
	D	10,710,1	10,610,2	23,310,3	23,2±0,4
30 days	F	10,910,1	10,310,6	23,810,8	23,8±1,0
	FD	10,610,2	11,010,7	23,410,3	24,1±0,5
	D	10,810,1	10,810,3	23,410,5	23,6±0,7
90 days	F	10,910,6	11,210,4	24,810,4	24,8±0,1
	FD	10,210,3	10,810,2	25,510,1	25,8±0,1
	D	10,710,0	10,410,0	24,310,3	23,6±0,3

AP = angular process, II = incisor insertion, IP = incisal point, SD = standard deviation; F = fractured group, FD = malnourished fractured group, D = malnourished group; LD = right side, LE = left side.

The Analysis of Variance showed a significant difference between the groups for the PA-II measurement: for the 90-day period, LE, with p= 0.027, and not significantly for the 24-hour periods, LD, with p= 0.440 and LE, with p= 0.436; for 7 days, LD, with p= 0.637 and LE, with p= 0.564; for 30 days, LD, with p= 0.113 and LE, with p= 0.564; for 7 days, LD with p= 0.637 and LE with p= 0.563; for 15 days, LD with p= 0.113 and LE with p= 0.564; for 30 days, LD with p= 0.077 and LE with p= 0.169 and for 90 days, LD with p= 0.213. Tukey's test or Dunnett's test identified the groups that differed from each other at 90 days, LE, there was no significant difference in the FD x F group, with p= 0.442 and FD x D, with p = 0.121 and F x D, with p= 0.158. Using the Friedman test, there was no significant difference between groups FD, LD, with p = 0.102 and LE, with p= 0.692, group F, LD, with p= 0.692 and LE, with p= 0.354 and group D, LD, with p= 0.792 and LE, with p= 0.187. When applying the *Student's t-test* for paired data to check for possible differences between the sides, there was a statistically significant difference for the FD group in the 15-day period LD x LE, with p= 0.037 and 90 days, LD x LE, with p= 0.010 and there was no significant difference for the 24-hour periods, LD x LE, with p= 0.791; 7 days, LD x LE, with p= 0.889 and 30 days, LD x LE, with p= 0.296; for group F, there was no significant difference for the periods of 24 hours, LD x LE, with p= 0.349; 7 days, LD x LE, with p= 0.378, 15 days, LD x LE, with p= 0.921; 30 days, LD x LE, with p= 0.204 and 90 days, LD x LE, with p= 0.176. And for group D, there was also no significant difference for the periods of 24 hours, LD x LE, with p= 0.170; 7 days, LD x LE, with p= 0.138; 15 days, LD x LE, with p= 0.974; 30 days, LD x LE, with p= 0.311 and 90 days, LD x LE, with p= 0.137.

For the PA-PI' measure, the *Analysis of Variance* showed a significant difference between the groups, for the 90-day period, LD, with p= 0.006 and LE, with p < 0.001. 0.001 and was not significant for the 24-hour periods, LD, with p= 0.410 and LE, with p= 0.443; for 7 days, LD, with p= 0.119 and LE, with p= 0.766; for 15 days, LD, with p= 0.181 and LE, with p= 0.537; for 30 days, LD, with p= 0.639 and LE, with p= 0.683. *Tukey's test* or *Dunnett's test* identified the groups that differed from each other, with a significant difference in the 90-day period, LD, the FD x D groups with p= 0.022 and LE, the FD x F groups, with p= 0.004, FD x D, with p= 0.006 and F x D, with p= 0.017 and there was no significant difference in the FD x F groups, with p= 0.163 and F x D, with p = 0.296. Using the *Friedman test*, there was no significant difference between groups FD, LD, with p = 0.126 and LE, with p = 0.155, group F, LD, with p = 0.126 and LE, with p = 0.113 and group D, LD, with p = 0.080 and LE, with p = 0.483. Using the *Student's t-test* for paired data to check for possible differences between the sides, there was a statistically significant difference for the FD group in the 30-day period, LD x LE, with p= 0.036 and there was no significant difference for the 24-hour periods, LD x LE, with p= 0.659; 7 days, LD x LE, with p= 0.670 and 15 days, LD x LE, with p= 0.474 and 90 days, LD x LE, with p= 0.056; for group F, there was no significant difference for the 24-hour periods, LD x LE, with p= 0.199;

7 days, LD x LE, with p= 0.185, 15 days, LD x LE, with p= 0.093; 30 days, LD x LE, with p= 0.912 and 90 days, LD x LE, with p= 0.887. And for group D, there was a significant difference for the 90-day period, LD x LE, with p= 0.048 and there was no significant difference for the 24-hour periods, LD x LE, with p= 0.851; 7 days, LD x LE, with p= 0.365; 15 days, LD x LE, with p= 0.220 and 30 days, LD x LE, with p= 0.571.

5.6 Histological study of the TMJs

The histological sections of the TMJ region on the right side of the animals sacrificed according to group and experimental period are described below.

5.6.1 Fractured Group

5.6.1.1 24-hour period

Histological sections showed a condylar fracture, with medial displacement of the fragment. The articular disc was preserved and remained close to the condyle. Neutrophilic, serofibrinous and fibrinous-haemorrhagic exudate was found in the joint space. An acute inflammatory process was observed near the joint capsule, as well as in the adjacent muscles. There was viable bone in the stumps, with foci of necrotic tissue between the bone fragments and adjacent proliferating fibrous connective tissue.

5.6.1.2 Seven-day period

Histological sections showed a fractured condyle with displacement, and the articular disc was positioned next to the condyle. One specimen showed areas of synovial membrane hyperplasia in the joint spaces. There was cartilaginous and bony proliferation around the fracture trace, with signs of resorption near the stumps. Interposed granulation tissue between the stumps, oedema and foci of necrosis in adjacent muscle tissue were observed.

5.6.1.3 15-day period

Histological sections revealed a fractured condyle with displacement and signs of remodelling. There was fibrous connective tissue and granulation in the joint spaces. Areas of necrosis in the bone stumps and bone callus formation (Figure 2-A) at the fracture site were observed.

5.6.1.4 30-day period

Histological sections revealed a remodelled and repositioned condyle with an interposed disc. One specimen showed a thickened articular disc with areas of chondrocyte clustering. There was exuberant bone callus next to the stumps, as well as areas of resorption and remodelling. Areas of cartilage (Figure 2-B) replaced by bone with the presence of osteoid material and osteoclasts next to the stumps were observed.

5.6.1.5 90-day period

Histological sections revealed a normal condylar process centred in the mandibular fossa, with an interposed articular disc. Re-modelling was observed in the mandibular ramus region, with remnants of bone callus in one specimen. Another specimen showed fibrocartilage atrophy with an area of resorption and remodelling on the condylar surface, with a thickened articular disc. There were no signs of an inflammatory process.

5.6.2 Malnourished Fractured Group

5.6.2.1 24-hour period

Histological sections revealed a condylar fracture with medial displacement. The articular disc was interposed and positioned, with oedema in the joint capsule. There was neutrophilic exudate and red blood cells in the joint space and adjacent muscles. Serofibrinous exudate was present between the stumps and an acute inflammatory process was observed in the upper and lower joint space and between the stumps. The stumps were devitalised, with reduced medullary spaces in the condyle and areas of resorption in the neck.

5.6.2.2 Seven-day period

Histological sections revealed a condylar fracture with displacement, with the articular disc positioned next to the condyle. There were areas of neoformed bone from the outer cortex of the stumps, with signs of resorption and devitalised areas next to the stumps. An inflammatory infiltrate was observed intramuscularly, in the capsule and also near the stumps.

5.4.1.1 15-day period

Histological sections revealed a condylar fracture with medial displacement. There was an intense intramuscular inflammatory and bone infiltrate. Areas of necrosis in the bone stumps and bone neoformation at the fracture site were observed. In one specimen there was resorption of the condyle, and in another the presence of bone sequestration.

5.4.1.2 30-day period

The histological sections showed signs of condylar atrophy with areas of re-modelling and resorption, with bone neoformation next to the stumps, also in the articular fossa. The fracture was not consolidated in two specimens, and one specimen showed bone sequestration with resorption of the condylar neck. The joint space was filled with fibrous connective tissue, with absence or remnants of articular fibrocartilage in the condyle, and the articular disc was not visible, suggesting fibrous ankylosis in all the animals in this group. An inflammatory process was observed around the fracture and in the adjacent muscle tissue.

5.6.2.5 90-day period

Histological sections revealed a remodelled condyle and ramus, with an interposed articular disc and areas of adherence to the condyle in two animals, with a picture suggestive of fibrous ankylosis. The condyle showed signs of atrophy in two animals and the articular fossa was remodelled. In one specimen, there was no consolidation of the fracture, resulting in pseudo-arthrosis.

5.6.3 Malnourished Group

5.6.3.1 24-hour and 7-day periods

Histological sections showed a normal condylar process, centred in the mandibular fossa and interposed by the articular disc. The articular surface of the condyle showed normal characteristics, covered by the articular surface, followed by the proliferative zone and fibrocartilage, as well as lamellar subchondral bone with medullary spaces.

5.6.3.2 15, 30 and 90 day periods

Histological sections showed a normal condylar process, centred in the mandibular fossa and interposed by the articular disc. The articular surface of the condyle was covered by the articular surface, followed by the proliferative zone and fibrocartilage, as well as lamellar subchondral bone with medullary spaces. Signs of fibrocartilage atrophy, with fewer chondrocytes, were observed in all the animals.

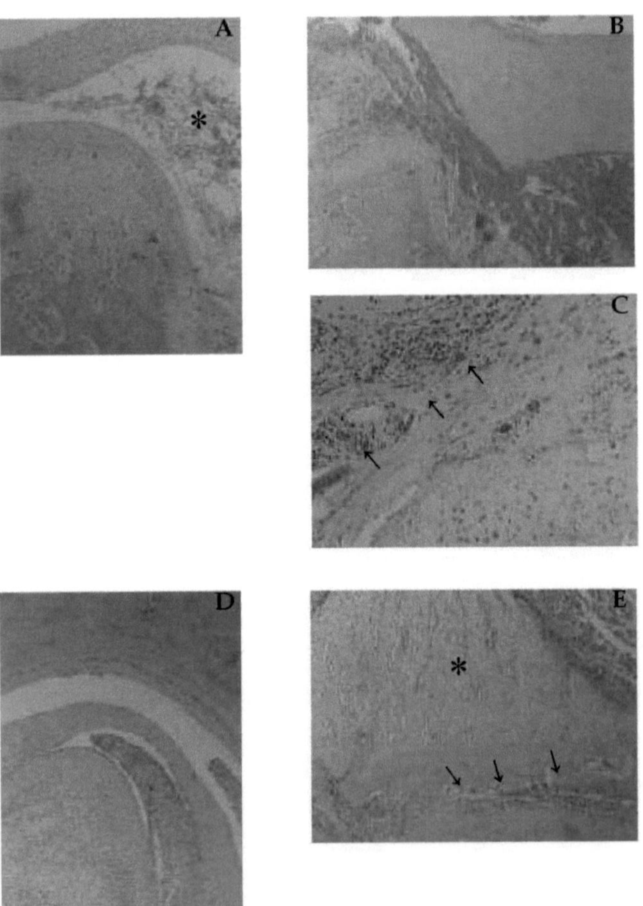

Figure 5.1 - Fractured Group. A = 24 hours - Presence of serofibrinous and fibrinohaemorrhagic exudate in the joint space (*)(40x). B = 24 hours - Detail of the fracture site, showing viable stumps

(40x). C = 24 hours - Neutrophilic exudate near the joint capsule (arrows) (100x). D = 7 days - Areas of synovial membrane hyperplasia in the supra- and infradiscal joint spaces (40x). E = 7 days - Area of intense bone neoformation (*), as well as signs of resorption near the bone stump (arrows) (40x).

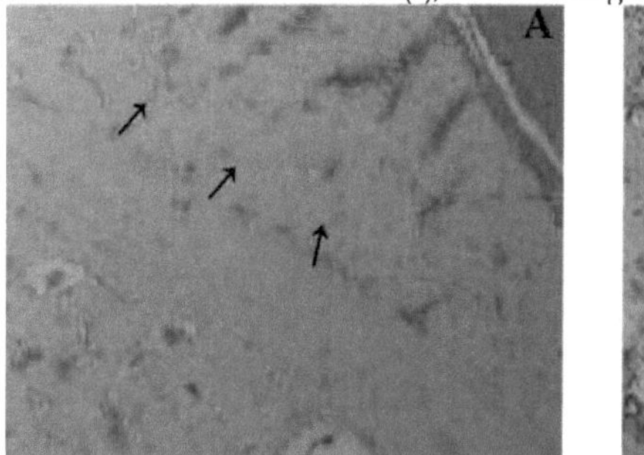

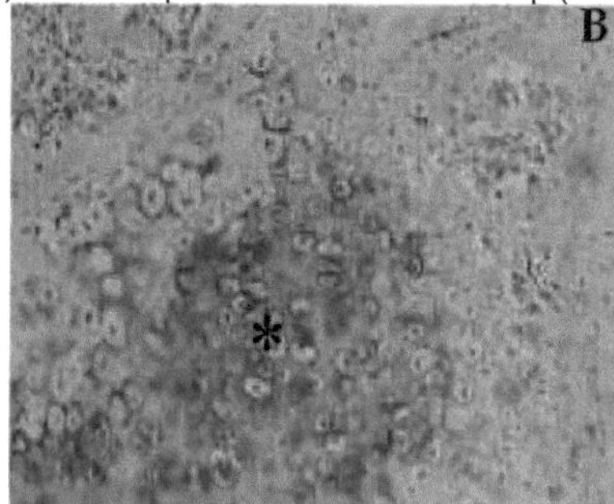

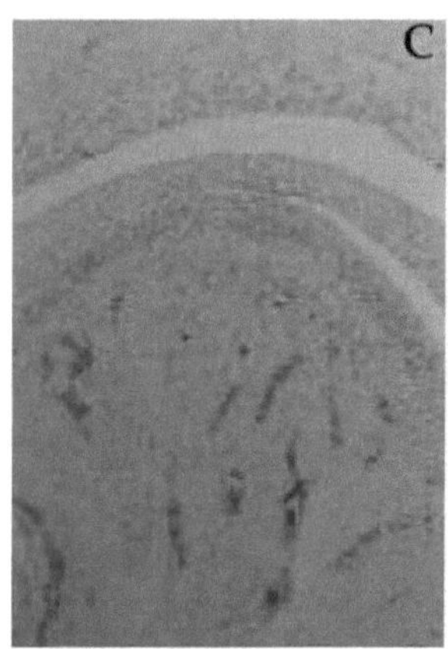

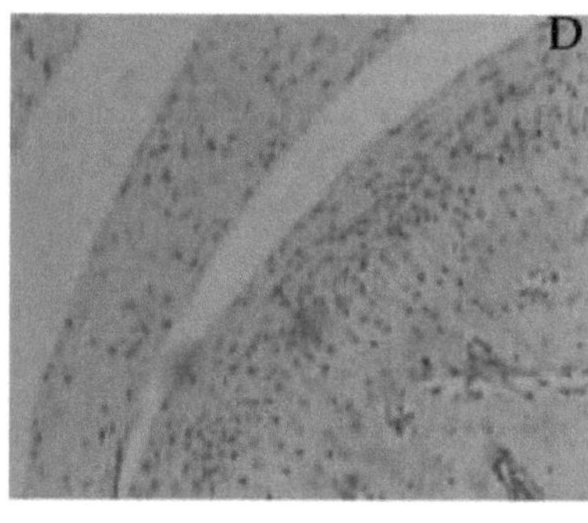

Figure 5.2 - Fractured Group. A = 15 days - Area of bone neoformation from the cortex of the bone stump (arrows) (40x). B = 30 days - Focal area of cartilage inside the bone callus is seen (*) (40x). C and D = 90 days - Condyle centred in the mandibular fossa, with interposed articular disc. C (40x) and D (100x)

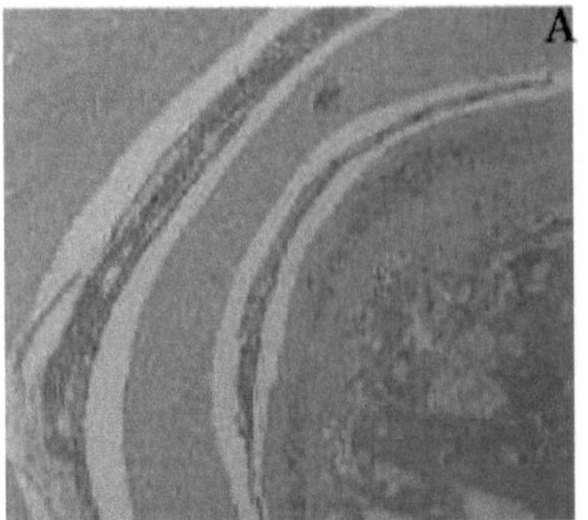

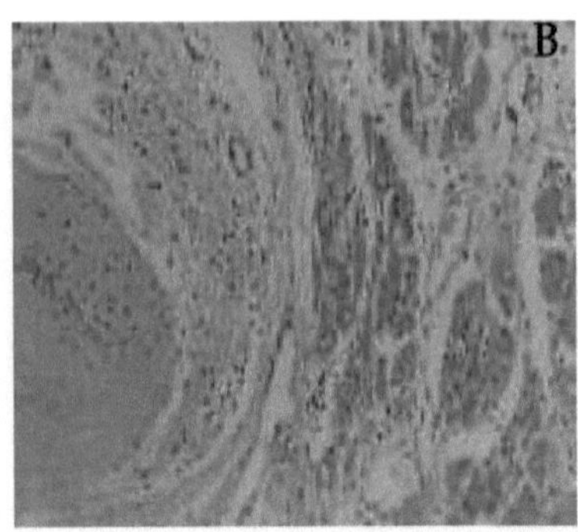

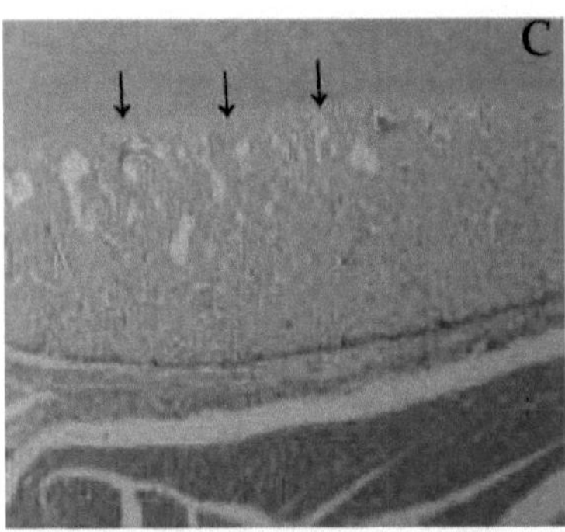

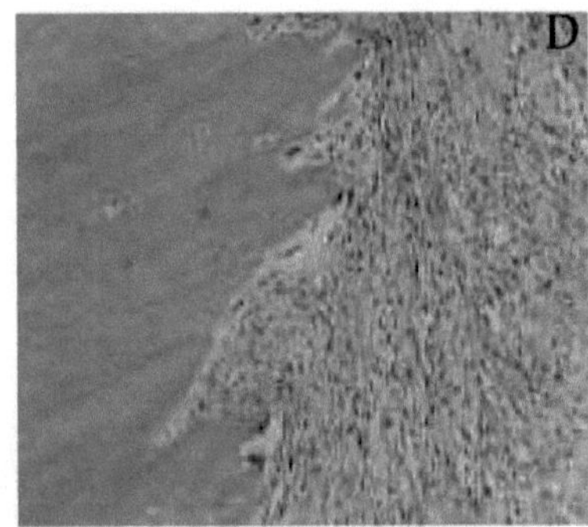

Figure 5.3 - Malnourished Fractured Group. A = 24 hours. Fibrmohaemorrhagic exudate in the supra- and infradiscal joint spaces (40x). B = 24 hours. Neutrophilic exudate near the capsule and associated musculature (100x). C = seven days. Area of neoformed bone from the external cortex of the bone stump (arrows) (40x). D = seven days. Detail of devitalised stump, with signs of resorption (100x).

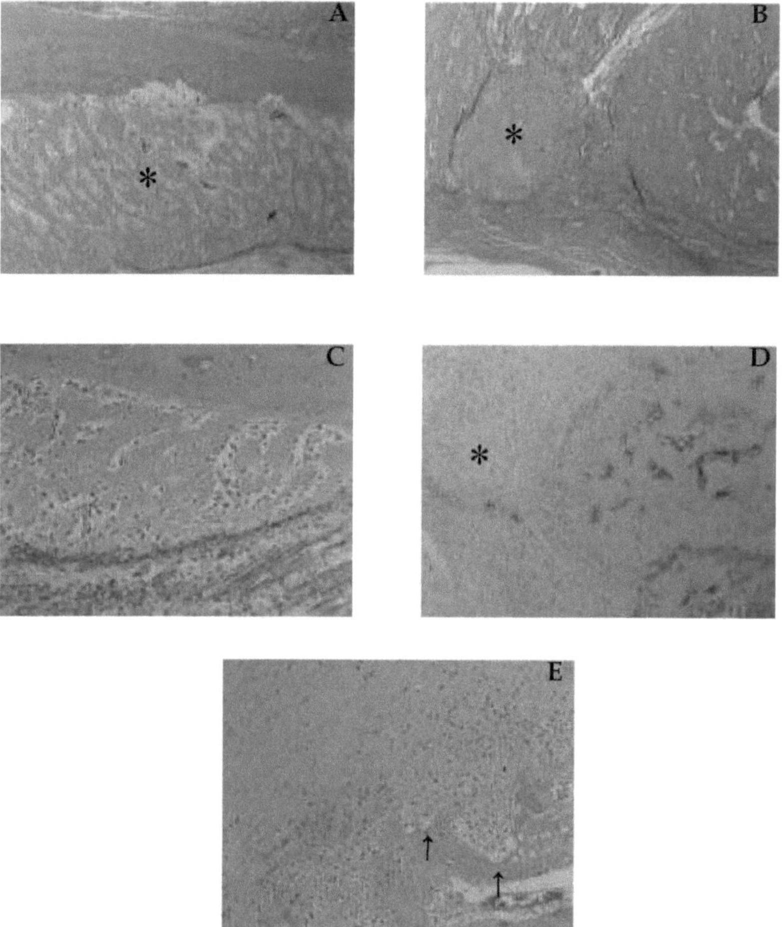

Figure 5.4 - Malnourished Fractured Group. A = 15 days - Area of intense bone neoformation (*) associated with areas of resorption (40x). B = 30 days - Detail of the stumps area showing connective tissue between them (*) (40x). C = 30 days - Area of bone neoformation from the centre of the bone stump (100x). D = 90 days - Note the atrophic condyle, with an extensive area of connective tissue in the joint space (*) (40x). E = 90 days - Atrophic articular surface, with areas of bone resorption (arrows) in continuity with connective tissue filling the joint space (*) (100x).

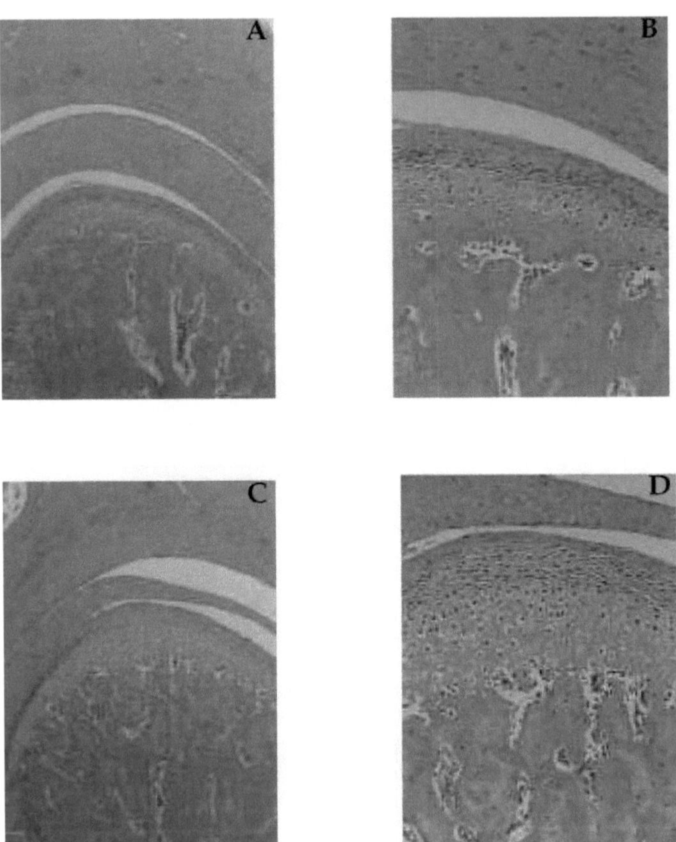

Figura 5.5 - Malnourished Group - Condylar process centred in the mandibular fossa, interposed by the articular disc. The articular cartilage of the condyle shows normal layers, as well as lamellar subchondral bone and medullary spaces. A = 24 hours (40x), B = 24 hours (100x), C = 7 days (40x), D = 7 days (100x)

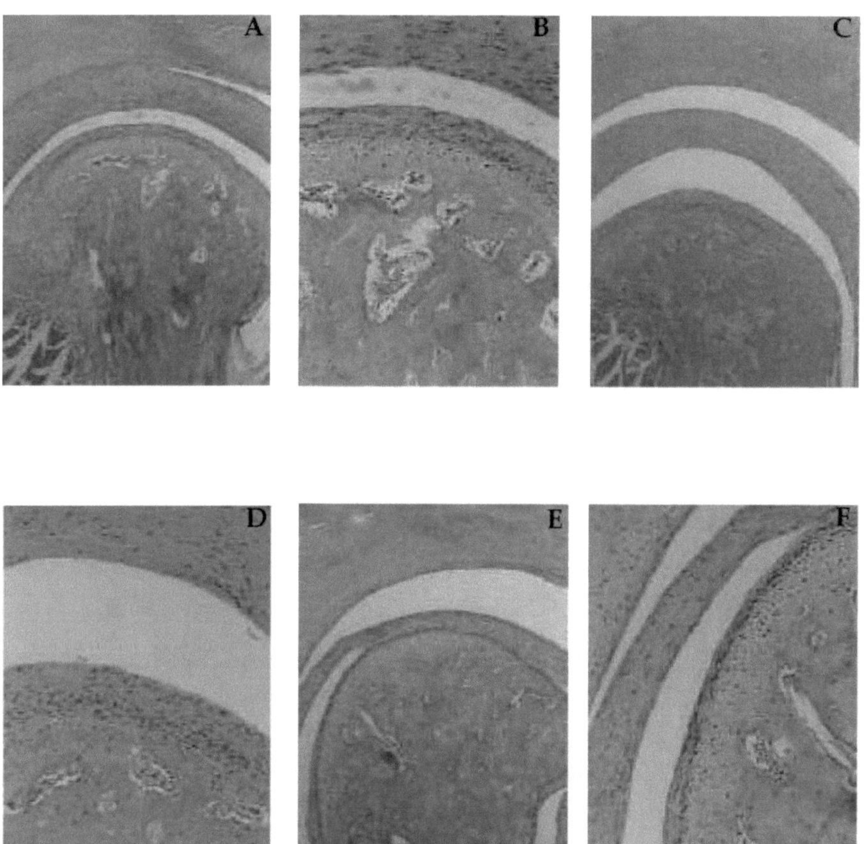

Figura 5.6 - Malnourished Group - Articular cartilage of the condyle covered by the articular surface, followed by the proliferative zone and fibrocartilage, lamellar subchondral bone and medullary spaces. Signs of fibrocartilage atrophy can be seen, with fewer chondrocytes. A = 15 days (40x), B = 15 days (100x), C = 30 days (40x), D = 30 days (100x), E = 90 days (40x), F = 90 days (100x)

CHAPTER 6

DISCUSSION

The repair of condylar fractures in rats subjected to a low-protein diet was assessed in adult rats. Feed, water and the coefficient of food efficiency were monitored, as well as body weight for comparative analysis of malnutrition. Blood biochemical and haematological tests were carried out to assess systemic changes in the face of malnutrition. To assess possible changes in fracture repair, cephalometric measurements were made using radiographs and a histological study of the fracture site and the TMJs. Using statistical tests, it was possible to identify the occurrence of macroscopic, symmetrical and biochemical alterations associated with condylar fractures in rats submitted to a hypoprotein diet. The changes in organic metabolism caused by trauma and surgery produce numerous problems related to protein, lipid and carbohydrate metabolism (MACHADO, 1993). Changes in the haemogram and blood biochemistry have been observed. In hospitalised patients with facial fractures, one study reported leucocytosis in 50% of cases, neutrophilia in 68% of cases and hyperglycaemia in 26.9% of the cases analysed (RODRIGUES; LUZ; MIORI, 1999). Another study showed a reduction in haemoglobin and haematocrit levels between the preoperative period and the 6-week postoperative period in patients undergoing orthognathic jaw surgery (LUZ; RODRIGUES, 2004).

Protein malnutrition is recognised as one of the main public health problems, as it can cause a significant increase in the incidence of mortality and morbidity in hospital environments (MACHADO, 1993; VANNUCCHI; UNAMUNO; MARCHINI, 1996). Many patients who develop protein-calorie malnutrition have been treated with a history of weight loss resulting from anorexia and increased catabolism associated with surgical catabolic trauma. The influence of protein malnutrition is present at all ages and can influence tissue regeneration (VANNUCCHI; UNAMUNO; MARCHINI, 1996). Even when an energy and protein diet is administered for 3 to 5 days after 6 days of trauma to elderly, malnourished patients hospitalised with lower limb fractures, it has been shown that they do not meet their energy and protein requirements (MILLER et al., 2006).

Malnutrition can result from inadequate nutrient intake as a sequel to diseases that lead to problems with ingestion, chewing, swallowing, digestion and absorption (AUN, 1997). Often, 30% to 50% of hospitalised patients have difficulty swallowing due to obstruction of the digestive tract, resulting from facial fractures, mainly mandibular, with moderate to severe malnutrition in 30% of cases (MACHADO, 1993).

In an association between childhood fractures and poverty status, a population study found that children in underserved areas had a significantly higher rate of fractures than those in affluent areas (STARK; BENNET; STONE, 2002).

Bone healing consists of a complex series of cellular events that require a high rate of protein synthesis. Several studies have emphasised the importance of eutrophic nutritional status and a diet with adequate levels of protein for the prevention and consolidation of fractures.

Malnutrition impairs the immune response and often results in infection and even increased mortality, as it reduces the number and function of T lymphocytes and the immune response (PALLARO; ROUX; SLOBODIANIK, 2001). The use of supplements stimulates immunity and can result in a reduction in infections, especially in the elderly, low birth weight newborns and malnourished hospitalised patients (CHAN-DRA 1999, 2002). Therefore, a patient's nutritional status is an important factor to be assessed in oral and maxillofacial surgery, because if there is a nutritional deficiency, it can be treated preoperatively with a balanced diet and supplements, as well as maintaining adequate protein intake postoperatively (CHIDYLLO;
CHIDYLLO, 1989). Malnutrition is common in hospitalised patients with fractures and contributes to delayed fracture healing, with increased morbidity (HUGHES et al., 2006). Protein malnutrition induces a decrease in resistance in the ileum and distal colon associated with a decrease in tissue collagen in the intestinal wall of rats (NAKAJIMA et al., 2008).

It has been observed radiographically that the effect of protein malnutrition on the evolution of bone repair in rat fractures in the growth and adult phases was not significant, as there was only evidence of faster bone repair in young rats and a delay in the evolution of bone callus in adult rats (RODRIGUES; ZUCAS, 1991). In another study, it was found that animals fed a low-protein diet and subjected to femur fractures produced callus composed of fibrous tissue, with a reduction in periosteum and a reduction in strength and hardness (DAY; DEHEER, 2001). Also, rats subjected to tibial fractures on a high-protein diet did not show fracture healing, but intermediate healing with fibrous tissue, unlike the group on a high-protein diet, which favoured the healing of experimental fractures by improving the organic quantity of the bone callus (GUARNI- ERO et al., 2003). In another experimental study on tibial fractures, it was observed that the formation of bone callus is normal, with regular tissue, in animals on a normal or hypoprotein diet with renutrition. However, it was observed that in animals on a low-protein diet there was fibrous tissue formation and less bone tissue formation (GUARNIERO et al., 1992). In newborn animals fed a low-protein diet, the jaws show satisfactory calcification compared to long bones, but there is a significant reduction in the amount of collagen produced (NAKAMOTO; MILLER, 1979a,b). However, there is no change in the concentration of protein and calcium (NAKAMOTO; MILLER, 1979a). The same has been seen in newborns whose mothers suffered malnutrition during pregnancy (NAKAMOTO; POR-TER; WINKLER, 1983), a reduction in growth, with changes in macrophage function, is described (PRESTES-CARNEIRO et al, 2006). In the post-natal period, the offspring of females with protein malnutrition showed bone morphological alterations, with reduced growth and alterations characteristic of delayed development, with a significant reduction in the number of cells in mitosis (BOLDRINI, 2003). However, it has been found that mineralisation is reduced due to insufficient degradation of proteoglycans in the mandible of protein-restricted animals (MIWA et al., 1989). When a protein-free diet with 20% casein is used, there is a reduction in the weight and thickness of the mandible, changes in mandibular bone proportions and deformities (ALIPPI et al., 1984). An experimental study using animals with protein malnutrition who underwent femoral fracture showed that subsequent renutrition with supplementary diets in the post-surgical phase had anabolic effects, with an increase in bone mineralisation, body mass and muscle mass (HUGHES et al., 2006).

However, the amount of protein that should be supplemented in the diet of post-surgical patients is uncertain, and the expected risks of complications from lower than necessary supplies are high, as is the risk of higher supplies (POMPEO, 2007).

To carry out the experiment, we used Wistar rats (Rattus norvegicus). The rat has been the animal of choice because it is small and easy to handle. It has been used to assess the repair process and the consequences for facial growth of injuries such as condylectomy or fractures of the mandible or condyle (GILHUUS-MOE, 1971; GRANSTROM; NILSSON, 1987; LIVNE; SILBERMANN, 1990; LUZ; ARAÚJO, 2001; RODRIGUES; LUZ, 2001; SHIMAHARA et al, 1987; SPRINZ, 1970; TEIXEIRA et al., 1998; YASUOKA; OKA, 1991).

Experimental mandible fractures represent a model that provides data similar to that found in the human skeleton. The fractures heal quickly, without major complications (GRANSTROM;

NILSSON, 1987). Bone changes related to the acute and chronic phases can be easily verified in this animal model (GRANSTROM; NILSSON, 1987). In the case of condylar fractures, this phenomenon is due to the man- dibular condyle's intense capacity for adaptation, as the condylar growth zone makes an important contribution to remodelling the TMJ after a fracture with displacement of this structure (GILHUUS-

MOE, 1971). It is interesting to note that the condyle fracture allows for the consumption of food during the experiment, allowing the animal to be maintained during the study period (LUZ; ARAÚJO, 2001; TEIXEIRA et al., 1998). This model also makes it possible to assess possible asymmetries in the maxilla and mandible by measuring radiographic images (GOULART et al., 1998; ROCHA et al., 1999; YAMAMO- TO; NOVELLI; LUZ, 1997).

The use of rats is also viable in studies aimed at bone repair in long bone fractures (CAMPOS, 2001; GUARNIERO et al., 2003; RODRIGUES; ZUCAS, 1991). The model also makes it possible to collect blood to determine biochemical markers and haematological tests (COSTA et al., 2000).

Alterations resulting from trauma to the TMJ are common (LINDQVIST et al., 1986; PROFFIT; VIG; TURVEY, 1980; SILVENNOIENEN et al., 1992). Of trauma to the TMJ, condylar fractures account for 52.4% of mandibular fractures (SILVENNOIENEN et al., 1992). Case studies have highlighted this fact (LARSEN; NIELS- EN, 1976; LINDQVIST et al., 1986). In terms of the location of condylar fractures, 71.5% were unilateral and of these, 19% were displaced and 81% were non-displaced (ANDERSSON; HALLMER; ERICKSSON, 2007; SILVENNOIENEN et al., 1992).

In this study, we used the unilateral condyle fracture with medial deviation as the surgical procedure. This is the most common form of condylar fracture (SILVENNOIENEN et al., 1992; MANGANELLO-SOUZA; LUZ, 2006). The realisation of unilateral experimental condylar fractures with medial deviation is in line with what occurs most frequently in patients. Condylar fractures most often occur in isolation, without the presence of other fractures (AMARATUN- GA, 1987; BELLI et al., 1987; TAKATSUKA et al., 2005). The unilateral form accounts for the majority of cases of this fracture (AMARATUNGA, 1987; BELLI et al., 1987; LINDQVIST et al., 1986). In these fractures, the condylar fragment often deviates medially (LINDAHL, 1977; WINSTANLEY, 1984).

When it comes to studying the TMJ, it's worth remembering that the articular layers are very similar to those of human beings. In addition, the relatively simple access to the TMJ facilitates the reproducibility of the experiment. The condyle and mandibular fossa are made up of cancellous bone covered by compact bone. The articular surfaces are covered by fibro-cartilage and the disc is made up of dense, avascular connective tissue. The joint capsule is formed by an external fibrous portion and the synovial membrane. In rats, the bone that presents the excavated mandibular fossa is the squamous bone, an independent bone in rodents, which in humans is joined to others to form the temporal bone. In this animal, the wall of the mandibular fossa is thicker than in humans, and the articular disc has few chondroid elements. It therefore constitutes a joint that is functionally compatible with the human TMJ (LIVNE; SILBERMANN, 1990; LUZ et al., 1991).

In this experimental condyle fracture model, it is possible to assess two aspects that occur simultaneously: the repair of the fracture itself and the remodelling of the TMJ, whether or not it recovers its original characteristics (GILHUUS-MOE, 1971; LUZ; ARAÚJO, 2001; TEIXEIRA et al., 1998).

Histologically, the articular surfaces are covered with fibrocartilage. The condyle has the following layers: articular surface or fibrous zone, proliferative zone, fibrocartilage, ossification zone and subchondral bone. The articular surface is made up of interlocking collagen bundles; the proliferative zone is thin; the fibrocartilage corresponds to growth cartilage; the ossification zone has trabeculae in formation; and the subchondral bone corresponds to the part with the largest volume. The articular disc is composed of collagen bundles and chondroid cells, making up fibrocartilage (LIVNE; SILBERMANN, 1990; LUZ; ARAÚJO, 2001; LUZ et al., 1991; TEIXEIRA et al., 1998). The cartilage of the mandibular condyle differs from primary cartilage in the morphological organisation of the chondrocytes and the response to biomechanical stress and humoral factors (ZHENG et al., 2005).

The conventional and hypoprotein diets were offered ad libitum. The hypoprotein feed proved to be effective in inducing a state of malnutrition, as verified by analysing blood biochemistry values. Analysing blood biochemistry can identify a state of malnutrition (DE LEEUW; VANDEWOUDE; VAN ELST, 1991). However, it was observed that the fractured group had a reduction in consumption in the immediate post-operative period, with recovery in the following periods. The reduction in feed intake observed is probably due to the difficulty in chewing in the post-operative period, associated with the stiffer texture of conventional feed when compared to cornstarch-based feed, which was softer. In another experimental study with rats, an increase in feed consumption with molasses supplementation was observed in the face of protein malnutrition

(COSTA et al., 2000).

In this study using hypoprotein feed, with a reduction in protein content from 23% to 8%, malnutrition was induced with a reduction in total protein and albumin. Similar findings were reported in an experimental study that used the same type of feed for a compatible period of time (ZANIN, 2003).

In the pre-clinical period of malnutrition, there are already biochemical changes that induce functional anatomical alterations, which depend on the organic reserves of nutrients and the adaptive metabolic changes that try to make up for the deficiency (NÓBREGA, 1998). On the other hand, despite the changes in protein levels due to the addition of starch, the concentrations that remained were probably able to prevent more serious clinical manifestations of malnutrition (ARAÚJO et al., 2003 a,b).

Water was also offered ad libitum. However, no water was consumed in the immediate post-operative period, between 24 hours and 7 days, in the fractured group, probably due to the surgical trauma. There was greater consumption in the malnourished fractured group, in most periods, probably due to their weakened general state as a result of the malnutrition associated with the post-operative period, which led to significant metabolic changes in these animals.

The coefficient of feed efficiency (CEA) evaluates the body weight gain of the animal fed a specific diet during the test period, as well as the efficiency of the feed as a whole. It has been used in various studies (COSTA et al., 2000; ORTEGA-FLORES et al., 2003; PELLET; YOUNG, 1980; RIBEIRO PASSOS DE OLIVEIRA et al., 2001; SGARBIERI, 1996). To assess the EAA in this study, the animals were weighed at the start of the experiment, at the time of the fracture and at sacrifice, and feed consumption was measured every 7 days by the difference between the food offered and the residual food. The EAA was obtained from the ratio between total weight gain and feed consumption during the experiment (CAMPBELL, 1963).

The CEA assessment showed a drop at the start of the experiment for all groups, and the fractured group showed a negative value at 24 hours; at 15 days there was a drop compared to the 7-day period. In this case, the animals ingested practically the same amount on average as they had in 7 days, but they lost weight compared to the 7-day group. In the malnourished group, there was a more or less constant intake of feed, but there was an increase in weight. In the malnourished fractured group there was a substantial weight loss, but food consumption was higher on average when compared to the other groups. This ratio recovered at the end of the experiment for all groups, indicating a return to normality.

Assessment of the animals' body weight in this study revealed that the fractured group showed a loss of weight in the immediate post-operative period, probably due to difficulty in swallowing. Progressive weight gain was observed after 7 days, with recovery at 90 days. Similar data, with a reduction in body weight but recovery by the end of the experiment, was observed in animals submitted to condylar fractures (LUZ; ARAÚJO, 2001; SHIMAHARA et al., 1987; TEIXEIRA et al., 1998; THALLER; REAVIE; DANILLER, 1990). It has also been found that animals subjected to indirect trauma to the TMJ or intra-articular injury show progressive weight gain (LUZ et al., 1991; PORTO; VASCONCELOS; SILVA JUNIOR, 2008). A study of condylar fractures, associated or not with intermaxillary block, found that the five-week block was related to weight gain deficiency (SHIMA-HARA; ONO; NAKANO, 1985). Another study involving condylar fractures in adult rats found statistically significant weight gain after 90 days in relation to the initial weight (TEIXEIRA et al., 1998). However, none of these authors used a control group for a more detailed assessment.

In our study, the animals in the malnourished group gained weight in all periods, probably due to the fact that the hypoprotein diet administered was rich in carbohydrates. Animals submitted to a hypoprotein diet (8%) and restricted B vitamins showed weight gain after 120 days due to the accumulation of fat from the excess carbohydrates in the diet (SANTANA; MOLINARI; MIRANDA NETO, 2001). However, in another study under the same conditions as the previous one, weight loss was observed (ZANIN, 2003). In a population study with malnourished children, it was observed that during the growth phase there is a loss of weight, but with an increase in the mass of fat deposited in the abdominal region, when compared to the control group (HOFFMAN, et al., 2007). It has been suggested that the accumulation of body fat is intended to promote a positive energy balance (JONES; SIMSON; FRIEDMAN, 1984). In this study, the animals in the malnourished fractured group lost weight at 7 and 15 days, with recovery and gain at 30 and 90 days. This longer time for weight recovery was probably due to malnutrition, which caused a significant metabolic change in these animals associated with the fracture, which was reflected in their weight. These results suggest an association between malnutrition with metabolic effects and condylar fracture, which compromised feeding. However, studies using animals on a high-protein diet and subjected to tibial fractures showed that there was weight loss until the end of the experiment (GUARNIERO et al., 2003; OLIVEIRA, 2003). In another study evaluating the effects of protein malnutrition on the intestinal wall in rats, there was also weight loss by the end of the experiment (NAKAJIMA et al., 2008).

Facial fractures, especially mandibular fractures, cause patients to lose weight due to difficulty chewing. However, studies have shown that, regardless of the surgical techniques used, this weight loss decreases as the fracture heals (KAPLAN; HOARD; PARK, 2001; THALLER; REAVIE; DANILLER, 1990). Nutritional changes resulting from this difficulty in eating have not been established.

In this study, it was observed that the reduction in weight can be attributed not to a lower food intake, since there was no significant drop in CEA, except in the malnourished fractured patient over the 7-day period, but rather to the injury and its repair process. In a study of patients with mandibular fractures, a group with immediate mobilisation and another group with immobilisation for a fortnight were assessed afterwards and the authors found that there was no significant difference between the groups, only weight loss and trismus for the immobilised group, probably due to the difficulty in swallowing associated with the surgical trauma and the repair process (KAPLAN; HOARD; PARK, 2001). However, the histological sections revealed an intense repair process in the fractured group, associated with an initial weight loss followed by progressive gain, which allows us to conclude that weight loss does not alter the repair dynamics. On the other hand, the malnourished fractured group showed weight loss and alterations in condylar repair. An experimental study promoting unilateral condylar fracture with deviation in rats maintained for one month by osteosynthesis showed an increase in the animals' weight (SHIMA- HARA et al., 1987). The reduced chewing ability and difficulty in swallowing experienced by patients with conventional complete dentures can make their diet deficient and thus increase the risk of malnutrition due to reduced food intake (OLIVEIRA; FRIGÉRIO, 2005). Another study looked at the relationship between dental status in elderly patients and nutritional status and found that edentulous patients had lower food intake (SHEIHAM et al., 2001). It is known that nutrition plays a role in bone growth and the prevention of classic deficiencies and that calcium intake can be an appropriate measure for bone growth and development (PRENTICE et al., 2006). However, it is known that an enriched protein diet in the immediate postoperative period in malnourished patients with fractures does not compensate for energy and protein needs (MILLER et al., 2006). Nutritional deficiencies should be checked preoperatively so that they can be treated with a balanced and supplementary diet, as well as maintaining adequate protein diet intake postoperatively (CHIDYLLO; CHIDYLLO, 1989).

These biochemical tests were carried out to detect possible systemic alterations that could justify malnutrition as a result of the difficulty in eating or the low-protein diet. A leucogram was also carried out in order to detect possible alterations due to the inflammatory process that had begun during the repair process.

Biochemical tests are used to assess nutritional status, both in experimentally induced alterations and in patients under various conditions and also under nutritional treatment (DE LEEUW; VANDEWOUDE; VAN ELST, 1981; HUGHES et al., 2006). For the biochemical analysis, blood (2 ml) was taken by cardiac puncture, in a similar way to another study (COSTA et al., 2000). Cardiac puncture is necessary due to the volume of blood to be obtained.

In order to assess nutritional status, it is necessary to determine a biochemical profile based on different parameters. Biochemical tests such as creatinine, serum transferrin, albumin and total lymphocyte count can help to identify malnutrition (DE LEEUW; VANDE-WOUDE; VAN ELST, 1981). It has also been reported that urea, complement C3, prealbumin and especially serum carotene can be included in the assessment of nutritional status in malnourished elderly patients (KERGOAT et al., 1987).

The negative control and reference values (MITRUKA; RAWNSLEY, 1977) were used to identify the clinical importance of the values obtained. Normal values in experimental models can vary according to the environment, strain, age of the animal, vivarium conditions and procedures carried out. The negative control was in line with the global limit presented by Mitruka and Rawnsley (1977), particularly the average serum albumin and alkaline phosphatase levels were below these values, but very close to the minimum limit.

Total proteins in the fractured group did not change significantly, but showed higher values when compared to the others, probably due to the high metabolic rates seen in the fracture healing process. The total protein values of the malnourished group remained within the minimum values compared to the negative control and the reference values. Based on these results, the total protein values associated with those of serum albumin and the total leucocyte count led us to consider that the protein malnutrition model adopted in this experiment was mild. Even in malnourished animals that underwent fracture and were renourished with a protein diet and supplements, there was also an increase in total protein levels (HUGHES et al., 2006). The animals in the malnourished fractured group had a decrease in total protein, with values below those of the fractured group and the malnourished group, particularly in the 30-day period, which may indicate a different behaviour in protein metabolism in this group, probably associated with changes in malnutrition rates aggravated by the fracture. A similar finding occurred in experimental tibial fractures in malnourished rats, with lower serum total protein levels maintained until the end of the experiment (OLIVEIRA, 2003). In an experimental study carried out with a high-protein diet and tibial fractures, there was also a reduction in total protein levels (GUARNIEIRO et al., 2003). Thus, the total protein index was an important indicator of bone metabolism in the fracture repair process and as an indicator of malnutrition (KERGOAT et al., 1987; MITRUKA; RAWNSLEY, 1977; OLIVEIRA, 2003; ZANIN, 2003). However, in an experimental study carried out on the foetuses of rats under protein restriction, high levels of protein were found in the animals' mandibles (MIWA et al., 1989).

The highest albumin levels were observed in the fractured group, especially in the 24-hour period, which is a period of intense protein mobilisation in the acute phase of post-fracture inflammation. The increase in albumin can be explained by the inflammatory process caused by the fracture itself (BORYS et al., 2004). At 15 days there was a significant drop in this group, with a substantial increase at 30 days, which may confirm a tendency to consider this phase very critical for the fractured individual, with a reduction in weight and a drop in total proteins (BORYS et al., 2004; DWYER et al., 2005; OLIVEIRA, 2003). The lowest albumin levels occurred in the fractured group malnourished at 24 hours and 30 days, as well as in the group malnourished at 24 hours. These values indicated that induced malnutrition caused a reduction in albumin levels (MELLANBY et al., 2005; NAKAJIMA et al., 2008; OLIVEIRA, 2003; ZANIN, 2003). Among a group of hospitalised patients with open fractures of the lower limbs, 50% of whom were malnourished, who were assessed for soft tissue healing based on biochemical parameters, it was found that there was a delay in the healing process in patients who had low albumin levels (DWYER et al., 2005). A reduction in albumin levels was seen in women with hip fractures, reflecting a poor nutritional state and consequent reduction in vitamin D (LÊ BOFF et al., 2000). It is likely that the association between fracture and protein malnutrition has interfered with hormonal metabolism, increasing the plasma level of parathyroid hormone and reducing the concentration of vitamin D (LAING; FRASER, 2002; LÊ BOFF et al., 2000; MELLANBY et al., 2005). Enteropathies with protein loss can reduce intestinal absorption of vitamin D and lower plasma calcium concentration, with low albumin and calcium concentrations being detected (MELLANBY et al., 2005). Low albumin levels have also been observed in animals with a protein diet and tibial fractures (GUARNIERO, 2003). However, animals with protein malnutrition that underwent fracture with subsequent renutrition with a protein diet and supplements showed an increase in albumin after 6 weeks (HUGHES et al., 2006).

Bone repair is also associated with calcium and alkaline phosphatase indices, which are markers of bone changes, especially in formation (SEE-BECK et al., 2005). In this study, the fractured and malnourished groups had calcium levels close to the negative control and reference values. The only trend observed was a slightly higher peak at 7 days. In the fractured group, it was found that the fracture alone was not enough to alter calcium metabolism, nor the malnourished state of the malnourished group induced in the experiment. However, in the malnourished fractured group there was a reduction in all periods when compared to the others. It is likely that the increased level of catabolism due to the inflammatory process in fractures, particularly in malnourished individuals, interferes with calcium levels, leading to poor bone repair and delayed bone callus formation (NAKA- MOTO; MILLER, 1979b; OLIVEIRA, 2003). It has been observed experimentally that during bone callus formation there are changes in calcium and phosphorus levels that are proportionally inverse to those of alkaline phosphatase, which increases significantly (KOMMENOU et al., 2005). In another study, they also found a reduction in calcium levels in the jaws of foetus rats subjected to protein restriction (MIWA et al., 1989). A greater amount of calcium has been observed in the mandibles of newborn rats with a gestational history of malnutrition and also that bone metabolism in the different growth centres subjected to nutritional alterations showed different behaviour when considering the mandible and long bones (NA- KAMOTO; PORTER; WINKLER, 1983). It is known that during fracture repair in dogs, a slight reduction in calcium levels has been observed 24 hours after the fracture, with a return to normality after 20 days (MILLER et al., 2006). In this study, this trend was also observed in the fractured group. However, hypocalcaemia occurred in the malnourished fractured group during all periods of the experiment, differing from the other groups, probably because catabolism produced an intense inflammatory process, a sign of malnutrition, particularly interfering with serum calcium levels.

Poor bone repair, with delayed callus formation and altered mechanical properties, may be related to hypocalcaemia in animals with protein malnutrition and fracture (DAY; DEHEER, 2001;

GUARNIEIRO et al., 1992).

In this study, the alkaline phosphatase level increased at 30 days in the fractured group, a period in which the bone callus is well formed. In the malnourished fractured group, there was a peak increase in alkaline phosphatase at 7 days and a decrease at 30 days, below the negative control. We can see that in fractured patients, alkaline phosphatase values are high at 30 days and that malnutrition causes a reduction in these values during this period (OLIVEIRA, 2003). The malnourished group also showed a drop in alkaline phosphatase at 30 days when compared to the 15-day period, the highest rate in a group that showed values below the negative control throughout the experiment. As alkaline phosphatase is an indicator of osteoblastic activity during fracture repair, an increase in its values has been observed concomitant with the formation of bone callus, although it shows great variation between individuals (SEEBECK et al., 2005). Thus, the variation between groups may indicate different periods in the formation of bone callus (CAMPOS, 2001; KOMMENOU et al., 2005; OLIVEIRA, 2003). On the other hand, malnutrition was apparently not responsible for the change in alkaline phosphatase levels in the malnourished group.

Average serum iron levels were lowest in the fractured group compared to the other groups. The malnourished fractured group showed a significant drop after 15 days, during which time the animal also showed lower weight and CEA levels. Thus, it was observed that the fracture associated with protein malnutrition leads to changes in this rate, with recovery in 90 days. The malnourished group had an increase in serum iron levels at 7 days, with an immediate drop at 15 days. Thus, in an individual on a normoprotein diet, the fracture during this experimental period of major tissue destruction/construction has an important effect on the serum iron level, reducing it to values that are borderline to those considered normal. It was also observed that the fracture during the period of great nutritional difficulty, over 7 days, had a significant effect on serum iron levels, reducing them (De LEEUW; VANDEWOUDE; VAN ELST, 1981; DWYER et al., 2005; MITRUKA; RAWNSLEY, 1977). On the other hand, malnutrition was apparently not responsible for the change in serum iron levels in the malnourished group.

Creatinine increased over 30 days in the fractured group, in the malnourished group over 15 days and in the malnourished fractured group there was an increase over 7 days and an equal drop over 15 days. The malnourished group showed values that exceeded the negative control in practically all the experimental periods. Thus, the higher values in this group may be related to the great extent of the muscular alterations (De LEEUW; VANDEWOUDE; VAN ELST, 1981; MITRUKA; RAWNSLEY, 1977). A study of malnourished, hospitalised patients with open fractures found that soft tissue healing took less time when the creatinine index was normal (DWYER et al., 2005).

Surgical trauma causes changes in the body, and the variation and consequences depend on the intensity of the surgical injury. Laboratory tests can help assess the general condition of these patients. The global leukocyte count and the differential leukocyte count were carried out in sequence to characterise the inflammatory cell response during fracture repair. Protein malnutrition can lead to a significant reduction in the immune response in both newborns and adults (CHANDRA, 2002).

In this experiment, the overall leucocyte count showed no significant changes, with the exception of the 15-day experimental period, where higher values were observed in the fractured and malnourished fractured groups. These values can be interpreted as being inherent to the state of fracture in these groups since it is known that there can be an increase in the leucocyte count in fractured individuals (RODRIGUES; LUZ; MIORI, 1999). At the same time, the 7 and 15 day periods showed the lowest CEA values for the malnourished fractured group. From the numerical values presented for the global leucocyte count, it cannot be said that there was a direct interference of the CEA on the leucocytes, since the other periods showed either higher or lower values. However, it can be said that the 15-day period brings about significant metabolic changes in the animal, which varies greatly in terms of nutritional status, a fact that also interferes with the overall leucocyte count, also contributing to its great variation during the experiment.

At 90 days, it can be seen that practically all the groups had a leukocyte rate similar to and higher than the negative control group, with the exception of the fractured group, whose value was very close to that of the negative control. This trend of proximity to the control group observed in the fractured group was detected in all experimental periods, with the exception of 30 days after the fracture. It is worth mentioning that the non-reduction of peripheral leucocytes was also observed in experimental models using rats with protein malnutrition (PRESTES-CARNEIRO et al., 2006). There was no quantitative alteration, but immunodeficiency cannot be ruled out in the malnourished animals, since the repair alterations suggest changes in the defence system, especially phagocytosis. A study of rats undergoing protein malnutrition showed alterations in macrophage function (PRESTES-CARNEIRO et al., 2006).

Individual leucocyte counts are used to check the proportion of the different leucocyte populations. In malnourished individuals, lymphocyte deficiencies have been reported, both in number and cellular function, especially in the regulation of cell-mediated immunity. Consumption of a low-protein diet causes thymus atrophy in growing rats, with a reduction in total T-lymphocyte cells, concomitant with an increase in immature thymocytes, thus limiting the immune response (KONNO et al, 1993; PALLARO et al., 2001). Similar phenomena are observed in malnourished senile individuals. In this experiment, lower lymphocyte values were observed in the malnourished group at 30 and 90 days, with significant differences in relation to the fractured group. During this period, the animals in the malnourished group were in a state of chronic malnutrition, characterised by ingestion of a hypoprotein diet for 60 and 120 days respectively, as well as being older. The reduction in lymphocytes in these animals probably follows the trends of immunosuppression observed in malnourished senile individuals, but more studies, especially involving thymic function, are needed to confirm these findings.

Lymphocytes were the most frequent cells in all groups and experimental periods. In normal, adult rats, the frequency of lymphocytes is higher than that of neutrophils (SANDERSON; PHILIPS, 1981).

The significant changes in the 24-hour and 7-day periods in the fractured and malnourished groups indicate that the condylar fracture interferes significantly with the leukocyte proportions. These periods can therefore be considered to represent the acute phase of inflammation during tissue repair, when a large number of polymorphonuclear cells occur, mainly to eliminate necrotic debris. As the malnourished group maintained a practically constant proportion of neutrophils during the initial phases, and the malnourished fractured group showed a similar oscillation to the fractured group, it can be said that the fracture was a determining factor in these changes. A study of patients with facial fractures showed the occurrence of leucocytosis and neutrophilia in this group (RODRIGUES; LUZ; MIORI, 1999).

To measure possible changes in the maxilla and mandible, we used radiographic examination. Cephalometric measurements helped to verify alterations, reducing possible difficulties in macroscopic evaluations (LUZ ; ARAÚJO, 2001; RODRIGUES; LUZ, 2001; TEIXEIRA; TEIXEIRA; LUZ, 2006). Various authors have used them in different models (DAS; MEYER;

SICHER, 1965; GIANELLY; MOORREES, 1965; GOULART et al., 1998; ROCHA et al., 1999; YAMAMOTO; NOVELLI; LUZ, 1997). Points were used that were observable radiographically and that had as reference structures that were not influenced by the fracture. Measurements were made using a computerised system, with the image enlarged, which allowed for greater precision in the data obtained (GOULART et al., 1998; ROCHA et al., 1999; RODRIGUES; LUZ, 2001; YAMAMOTO; NOVELLI; LUZ, 1997).

In the axial view of the skull, measurements were made of the length of the maxilla and mandible and the angle "A" to determine deviation from the man- dibular midline (GOULART et al., 1998; LUZ; ARAÚJO, 2001; RODRIGUES; LUZ, 2001; YAMAMOTO; NOVELLI; LUZ, 1997).

In this study we found a deviation of the mandibular midline from the maxillary midline in the fractured and malnourished fractured groups for the 15-day period and a greater deviation in the malnourished fractured group for the 90-day period, with a highly significant difference. To determine this deviation, the "A" angle was measured. Using an axial view of the skull, a line was drawn immediately anterior to the tympanic bulla on the right and left sides and the median point was determined. Then, based on the point between the upper (PI) and lower (PI') incisors, the "A" angle was measured, allowing the deviation from the midline between the maxilla and mandible to be quantified (LUZ; ARAÚJO, 2001; RODRIGUES; LUZ, 2001; YAMAMOTO; NOVELLI; LUZ, 1997). In other experimental studies, the occurrence of asymmetries has been verified through macroscopic observations and cephalometric studies based on radiographs, making it possible to quantify these asymmetries (BOLDRINI, 2003; GIANELLY; MOORREES, 1965; LUZ; ARAÚJO, 2001; RODRIGUES; LUZ, 2001; TEIXEIRA; TEIXEIRA; LUZ, 2006). Bilateral condylar fractures require more extensive adaptations to the masticatory system, but have more favourable results compared to unilateral condylar fractures (ELLIS; TH- ROCKMORTON, 2005). It has been described that the altered condyle position affects the mandibular growth pattern, causing asymmetry (AYOUB; MOSTAFA, 1992). Although the condyle is considered to be the main growth centre of the mandible, muscular action or another type of force will be responsible for compensation in the absence of the condyle (KOSKI, 1968). The degenerative process has been observed radiographically in condyle fractures in young rats (TEIXEIRA; TEIXEIRA; LUZ, 2006).

In this study, there was a reduction in maxillary length on the right or fracture side, confirmed by the distance between the tympanic bulla and the infraorbital foramen at 90 days for the malnourished fracture group and between the infraorbital foramen and the maxillary incisal point at 15 days and 90 days for the malnourished fracture group. There was also a decrease in the length of the mandible, on the right or fracture side, confirmed by the distance between the angular process and the insertion of the mandibular incisor at 15 days and 90 days for the malnourished fracture group, and the angular process and the incisal point of the mandible at 30 days for the malnourished fracture group and 90 days for the malnourished group. Thus, it can be seen that the effects of condylar fracture in malnourished animals were greater in the occurrence of asymmetries, not only in the mandible but also in the maxilla. The role of dental occlusion has been demonstrated in facial growth, promoting an association between maxillary and mandibular growth. Thus, interference with mandibular growth, such as fracture or removal of the mandibular condyle, leads to a reduction in maxillary growth and vice versa (ENLOW et al., 1977; RODRIGUES; LUZ, 2001; TEIXEIRA; TEIXEIRA; LUZ, 2006). The influence of condylar fractures on the length of the maxilla and mandible has been verified by other authors in experimental studies, and a compensation in masticatory function by means of a neuromuscular mechanism could also influence this process (ENLOW et al., 1977; PROFFIT; VIG; TURVEY, 1980; TEIXEIRA; TEIXEIRA; LUZ, 2006).

Histological analysis of the TMJs and condylar processes showed articular alterations in all the experimental groups, as well as allowing a description of the fracture repair process in the groups where it was instituted. It is therefore worth recalling the histological characteristics of the TMJ.

The TMJ has fibrocartilage on the articular surfaces, which are interposed by a fibrocartilaginous disc. The condyle is made up of the following layers: the articular surface (fibrous zone), made up of collagen fibre bundles; the thin pro- liferative zone (mitosis zone); fibrocartilage (cartilaginous zone), represented by hyaline cartilage and subchondral bone (ossification zones), corresponding to the largest volume of the condylar structure. Histologically, the composition of the rat TMJ is similar to that of the human TMJ (LUZ et al., 1991; YASUOKA; OKA, 1991).

The histological findings after 24 hours in the fractured and malnourished fractured groups showed a condylar fracture, with medial displacement, presence of neutrophilic, serofibrinous exudate next to the fracture trace (LUZ; ARAÚJO, 2001). These aspects represent the initial phase of the inflammatory process in the face of a fracture (CORMACK, 1987). Experimental condyle fractures have also revealed this data (SHIMAHARA; ONO; NAKANO, 1985; TEIXEIRA et al.,

1998). The joint showed a preserved, interposed and positioned articular disc, with the presence of neutrophilic exudate and red blood cells in the joint space, with foci of necrotic tissue between the bone fragments and adjacent proliferating fibrous connective tissue. In the fractured group there was viable bone in the stumps, while in the malnourished fractured group the stumps were devitalised, with reduced medullary spaces in the condyle and areas of resorption in its neck. Few studies that have promoted experimental condyle fractures with deviation have shown that the articular disc accompanies the condyle, maintaining its association (PINKERT, 1982; TEIXEIRA et al., 1998). The other findings correspond to the inflammatory response to trauma (LUZ et al., 1991; TEIXEIRA et al., 1998). The presence of intra-articular bleeding after trauma is controversial in the literature. In this study, this finding seems to be related to the presence of the fracture. In a study that involved indirect trauma to the TMJ, no haemarthrosis was found (LUZ et al., 1991). On the other hand, a study using arthroscopy revealed that haemarthrosis is common in mandibular trauma (GOSS; BOSANQUET, 1990). It has been shown that experimental condyle fractures cause serofibrinous exudate in the joint space (LUZ; ARAÚJO, 2001; TEIXEIRA et al., 1998).

Histological data after 7 days revealed cartilaginous and bone proliferation around the fracture trace in the fractured group (LUZ; ARAÚJO, 2001). This finding corresponds to the beginning of bone callus formation, which is caused by the proliferative activity of the periosteum (CORMACK, 1987). In experimental mandibular fractures in rabbits or rats, a similar aspect is observed (CRAFT et al., 1974; GRANSTROM; NILSSON, 1987). There were signs of resorption in the stumps in our experiment. This contrasts with what was observed in experimental condyle fractures in adult rats, which showed areas of devitalised bone in the stumps, in parallel with the proliferation described (TEIXEIRA et al., 1998). However, in the malnourished fractured group, there was bone proliferation from the outer cortex of the stumps, which were devitalised, without the obvious presence of cartilage in its middle. The presence of an inflammatory infiltrate near the capsule, stumps and adjacent muscle tissue is expected as a consequence of trauma (LUZ et al., 1991; SHIMAHARA; ONO; NAKANO, 1985).

The histological findings after two weeks in the fractured group correspond to the proliferation of cartilaginous and bone tissue near the fracture stumps, resulting in local thickening. This finding comprises the phase in which the bone callus is formed and binds the fragments together (CORMACK, 1987). Experimental mandible fractures in rabbits and rats showed the same phenomenon during this period (CRAFT et al., 1974; GRANSTROM; NILSSON, 1987; MABUSHI, 1988). Also in other studies, the formation of exuberant bone callus was observed within 15 days (LUZ; ARAÚJO, 2001; LUZ et al., 1991; TEIXEIRA et al., 1998). In general, studies promoting experimental condyle fractures have described their repair through the formation of bone callus (BOYNE, 1967; SHIMAHARA; ONO; NAKANO, 1985; TEIXEIRA et al., 1998; YASUOKA; OKA, 1991). The presence of fibrous connective tissue and granulation in the joint spaces corresponds to the response to joint trauma (LUZ et al., 1991; SHIMAHARA; ONO; NAKANO, 1985). However, in the malnourished fractured group there was a persistent intramuscular inflammatory and bone infiltrate, and in one specimen there was resorption of the condyle, and in another, the presence of bone sequestration.

Histological data after 30 days showed a remodelled condylar process with an interposed articular disc in the fractured group. These data correspond to the normal characteristics described for the rat TMJ (LUZ; ARAÚJO, 2001), with the presence of exuberant bone callus within one month (TEIXEIRA et al., 1998) areas of resorption and remodelling with the presence of osteoid material and osteoclasts next to the stumps correspond to the final phase of repair through bone callus (CRAFT et al., 1974; BANKS; MACKENZIE, 1975; GRANSTROM; NILSSON, 1987; ZENG et al., 2005). In the malnourished fracture group, the fracture was not consolidated in two specimens, one specimen showed bone sequestration with resorption of the condylar neck and in all the animals the joint space was filled with fibrous connective tissue, with absence or remains of articular fibrocartilage in the condyle, without evidence of the articular disc, configuring a picture suggestive of fibrous ankylosis. Another study of indirect trauma to the TMJ noted the presence of fibrous adhesion after trauma (LUZ et al., 1991). There was also the presence of an inflammatory process in the

around the fracture and in the adjacent muscle tissue. These findings do not correspond to the sequential process expected for this period, probably associated with the malnourished state of the animals in this group. Other experimental studies with tibial fractures and a high-protein diet also found a case of fracture non-healing and intermediate healing, with fibrous tissue, in the rest of the group, 30 days after surgery (GUARNIERO et al., 1992, 2003).

The histological aspects observed after 90 days corresponded to normal characteristics of the condylar process, including its tissue components and their positioning in the fractured group (LUZ;

ARAÚJO, 2001).

Another study, which carried out condylar fractures with a deviation in adult rats, also found aspects of normality within three months (TEIXEIRA,et al., 1998). Experimental studies in rats have demonstrated the repair of condylar fractures without deviation, through the formation of bone callus. In this study, in the malnourished fracture group, one specimen showed remnants of bone callus. However, the literature is controversial in relation to the period required to complete the repair process, ranging from five weeks to two months (SHIMAHARA; ONO; NAKANO, 1985; SHIMAHARA et al., 1987). Even a study using young rats reported complete bone union within two months (YASUOKA; OKA, 1991). Osteoclastic activity was observed near the condyle, which corresponds to the remodelling process that occurs in the repair of condylar fractures. The authors are unanimous when describing the remodelling process observed in various experimental models, such as: condyle fracture without deviation (BANKS; MACKENZIE, 1975; BOYNE, 1967; SHIMAHARA; ONO; NAKANO, 1985; YASUOKA; OKA, 1991) condyle fracture with deviation (SHIMAHARA et al., 1987; TEIXEIRA et al., 1998); subcondylar os-theotomy (MONJE et al., 1993); indirect trauma to the TMJ (LUZ et al., 1991). This phenomenon is associated with the insertion of the lateral pterygoid muscle (BANKS; MACKENZIE, 1975).

Atrophy of the fibrocartilage are signs of a degenerative process with an area of resorption and remodelling on the condylar surface and an abnormal contour. This was observed in all groups, with one specimen from the fractured group, two specimens from the malnourished fractured group and all three specimens from the malnourished group after 90 days. This phenomenon has been described by some authors in the case of procedures such as condylar fractures treated in a crude or uncrude manner (AHMED et al., 1978); indirect trauma to the TMJ (LUZ et al., 1991); subcondylar osteotomy (MONJE et al., 1993) or theotomy with osteosynthesis and screw (SUURONEN et al., 1994). Basically, in this model of condylar fractures with deviation, this finding has been rare (TEIXEIRA et al., 1998). The degenerative process probably occurs due to an association of factors that may complicate the pre-existing trauma (MARKEY; POTTER; MOF- FETT, 1980). The ability of the condyle to adapt to traumatic injuries may also explain the rarity of the degenerative process. A series of studies have demonstrated this phenomenon, with activity through cartilage proliferation and areas of bone resorption (BANKS; MACKENZIE, 1975; BOYNE, 1967; GILHUUS- MOE, 1971; LUZ et al., 1991; SHIMAHARA et al., 1987; YASUOKA; OKA, 1991). However, an experimental study with young rats showed that condylar fractures repair normally but can lead to degenerative changes (TEIXEIRA; TEIXEIRA; LUZ, 2006). Condylar activity is described by the thickening of the proliferative zone or of the various layers that make up the articular fibrocartilage (GILHUUS-MOE, 1971; LUZ et al., 1991; MABUCHI, 1988). Condylar deformities occur when the displacement of the fragments is greater (TAKATSUKA et al., 2005).

In the malnourished fracture group, at 90 days, two animals showed that the disc was interposed with areas of adherence to the condyle, suggestive of fibrous ankylosis. In one of these specimens, the fracture was not consolidated, resulting in pseudo-arthrosis. In an experimental study on rats, removal of the articular disc induced the development of fibrous ankylosis within 90 days (PORTO; VASCONCELOS; SILVA JUNIOR, 2008).

The histological findings after 24 hours and 7 days in the malnourished group were normal. However, at 15, 30 and 90 days, the presence of fibrocartilage atrophy with an area of resorption and remodelling on the condylar surface was also observed in the malnourished group in all animals.

The aim of this study was to assess repair and indicators of malnutrition in rats subjected to unilateral mandibular condyle fractures and protein malnutrition, demonstrating the significant effects of this type of malnutrition on the fractured individuals. Groups of fractured, malnourished fractured and malnourished animals were formed and macroscopic, blood biochemical, cephalometric radiographic and histological evaluations were carried out, which allowed correlations between the factors to be established. The unilateral mandibular condyle fracture associated with protein malnutrition led to low food efficiency ratio values, negative changes in total protein, albumin and serum calcium values, leukocytosis, mandibular midline deviation, as well as compromised bone callus formation and induced fibrocartilage atrophy and fibrous ankylosis.

CHAPTER 7

CONCLUSIONS

In this study on the repair and malnutrition indicators of rats submitted to mandibular condyle fracture and protein malnutrition, it was possible to conclude that:

1. Feed and water consumption was higher in the malnourished fractured group in most periods.
2. CEA values were low, especially in the initial periods, and were more significant in the malnourished fractured group. There was little weight gain in the initial periods, except in the malnourished fractured group, which showed significant losses in this period, with weight gain in the other periods, significantly lower in the malnourished fractured group.
3. Blood biochemistry tests showed a drop, especially in the early periods, in total protein and albumin values, as well as in serum calcium in all periods, which was significant for the malnourished fracture group.
4. The leucogram showed an increase, especially in the early periods, in leucocytes, lymphocytes and neutrophils, which was more significant in the malnourished fracture group.
5. There was a significant deviation of the mandibular midline from the maxillary midline in the malnourished fractured group, as well as asymmetry of the maxilla and mandible, especially towards the end of the experiment.
6. Histological analysis showed that protein malnutrition led to atrophy of the condyle fibrocartilage. Fracture under malnutrition compromised bone callus formation and induced fibrocartilage atrophy and fibrous ankylosis.

REFERENCES

Ahmed MA, El-Mahdy A, Attia MA, El Rahman HA. Open reduction and interosseous wiring versus closed reduction and immobilisation in the treatment of condylar neck fractures during the growth period of the mandible in dogs.Egypt Dent J 1978; 24:431- 44.

Alippi RM, Barcelo AC, Bardi M, Friedman SM, Rio ME, Bozzini CE. Effect of protein- free diet on growth of the skeletal units of the rat mandible. Acta Odontol Latinoamer 1984;1:9-13.

Amaratunga NAS. A study of condylar fractures in Sri Lankan patients with special reference to the recent views on treatment, healing and sequelae. Br J Oral Maxillofac Surg 1987;25:391-7.

Andersson J, Hallmer F, Eriksson L. Unilateral mandibular condylar fractures: a 31 - year follow-up of non - surgical treatment. Int. J Oral Maxillofac Surg 2007;36:310-4.

Araújo EJA, SanfAna DMG, Molinari SL, Miranda-Neto MH. Effect of protein and vitamin B deficiency on the morphoquantitative aspects of the myenteric plexus of the descending colon of adult rats. Arq Neurops 2003a; 61:226-33.

Araújo EJA, SanfAna DMG, Molinari SL, Miranda-Neto MH. Regional differences in the number and type of myenteric neurons in the ascending colon of rats. Arq Neurops 2003b;61:220-5.

Aun F. Nutrition in surgery. In: Birolini D, Utiyama E, Steinman E. Cirurgia de emergência. São Paulo: Atheneu; 1997.

Ayoub AF, Mostafa YA. Aberrant mandibular growth: theoritical implications. Am J Orthod Dentofac Orthop 1992;101:255-65.

Banks P, Mackenzie I. Condylotomy. A clinical and experimental appraisal of a surgi- cal technique. J Maxillofac Surg 1975;3:170-81.

Belli E, Battistella G, Forti P, De Ponte F. Statistical evaluation of 85 patients affected by condylar fracture. Minerva Stomat 1987;36:883-90.

Boldrini, SC. Effects of pre- and post-natal protein malnutrition and post-natal renutrition on craniofacial growth in wistar rats: craniometric, morphoquantitative and ultrastructural analyses. Thesis [PhD]. São Paulo: USP Biomedical Sciences Institute; 2003.

Borys J, Grabowska SZ, Antonowicz B, Driyl D, Citko A, Rogowski F. Collagen type I and III metabolism in assessment of mandible fractures healing. Rocz Akad Med Bia- lymst 2004;49:237-45

Boyne PJ. Osseous repair and mandibular growth after subcondylar fracture. J Oral Surg 1967;25:300-9.

Campbell JA. Method for determination of PER & NPR. In: Committee on Protein Malnutrition. Food and Nutrition Board. Evaluation of protein quality. Washington; 1963. p. 31-2.

Campos WG. Evaluation of the effect of the ossein-hydroxyapatite complex on fracture healing in protein malnutrition. Experimental study in rats. Acta Ortop Bras 2001;9:21-5.

Chandra RK. Nutrition and immunology: from the clinic to cellular biology and back again. Proc. Nutrition Society 1999;58:681-3.

Chandra RK. Nutrition and the immune system from birth to old age. European J Clin Nutr 2002;56, suppl. 3:573-6.

Chidyllo SA, Chidyllo R. Nutritional evaluation prior to oral and maxillofacial sur- gery. N Y State Dent J 1989;55:38-40.

Cormack DH. Ham's histology. Philadelphia: JB Lippincott; 1987.

Costa M, Moraes L, Bion F, Rivera M, Moura L, Conceição M. Evaluation of the efficacy of molasses supplementation in the diet of normal and depleted rats. Arch Latinoam Nutr 2000;50:341-5.

Craft PD, Mani MM, Pazel J, Masters FW. Experimental study of healing in fractures of membranous bone. Plast Reconstr Surg 1974; 53: 321-5.

Das AK, Meyer J, Sicher H. X-ray and alizarin studies on the effect of bilateral con- dylectomy in the rat. Angle Orthodont 1965; 35:138-148.

Day SM, DeHeer DH. Reversal of the detrimental effects of chronic protein malnutri- tion on long bone fracture healing. J Orthop Trauma 2001;15:47-53.

De Leeuw I, Vandewoude M, Van Elst F. Nutritional assessment as a quality control of total parenteral nutrition. Acta Chir Belg 1981;80:145-8.

Dwyer AJ, John B, Mam MK, Antony P, Abraham R, Joshi M. Nutritional status and wound healing in open fractures of the lower limb. Int Orthop 2005;29:251-4.

Ellis E, Throckmorton GS. Treatment of mandibular condylar process fractures: Bio- logical considerations. J Oral Maxillofac Surg 2005;63:115-34.

Enlow DA, Harvold EP, Latham RA, Mofet BC, Christiansen RL, Hausch HG. Research on control of cranio facial morphogenesis: An NIDR State - of the Art Workshop. AJO- DO 1977;p.509-30.

Gianelly AA, Moorrees CFA. Condylectomy in the rat. Arch Oral Biol 1965; 10:101-6.

Gilhuus-Moe O. Fractures of the mandibular condyle in the growth period. Acta Odont Scand 1971;29:53-63.

Goss AN, Bosanquet AG. The arthroscopic appearance of acute temporomandibular joint trauma. J Oral Maxillofac Surg 1990;48:780-3.

Goulart AC, Fernandes EMV, Cavalcanti FC, Novelli MD, Luz JGC. Fracture of the zygomatic arch during growth. Experimental study in rats. Rev Odontol Univ São Paulo 1998;12:75-80.

Granstrom G, Nilsson LP. Experimental mandibular fracture: studies on bone repair and remodellation. Scand J Plast Reconstr Surg Hand Surg 1987;21:159-65.

Guarniero R, de Barros Filho TE, Tannuri U, Rodrigues CJ, Rossi JD. Study of fracture healing in protein malnutrition. Rev Paul Med 1992;110:63-8.

Guarniero R, Cinagava MY, Santana PJ, Batista MA, Oliveira LAA, Rodrigues CJ, Cinagava FT. Influence of the protein component on fracture healing: experimental work in rats. Acta Ortop Bras 2003;11:206-10.

Hoffman DJ, Martino PA, Roberts SB, Sawaya AL. Body fat distribution in stunted compared with normal - height children from the shantytowns of São Paulo, Brazil. Nutrition 2007;23:640-6.

Hughes MS, Kazmier P, Burd TA, Anglen J, Stoker AM, Kuroli K, et al. Enhanced fracture and soft-tissue healing by means of anabolic dietary supplementation. J Bone Joint Surg Am 2006;88:2386-94.

Jones AP, Simson EL, Friedman MI. Gestational under nutrition and the development of obesity in rats. J Nutr 1984;114:1482-84.

Kaplan BA, Hoard MA, Park SS. Immediate mobilisation following fixation of man- dible fractures: a prospective, randomized study. Laryngoscope 2001;111:1520-4.

Kergoat MJ, Leclerc BS, PetitClerc C, Imbach A. Discriminant biochemical markers for evaluating the nutritional status of elderly patients in long-term care. Am J Clin Nutr 1987;46:849-61.

Kommenou A, Karayannopoulou M, Polizopoulou ZS, Constantinidis TC, Dessiris A. Correlation of serum alkaline phosphatase activity with the healing process of long bone fractures in dogs. Vet Clin Pathol 2005;34:35-8.

Konno A, Utsuyama M, Kurashima C, Kasai M, Kimura S, Hirokawa K. Effects of a protein -free diet or food restriction on the immune system of Wistar and Buffalo rats at different ages. Mech Ageing Dev 1993;72:183-97.

Koski KL. Cranial growth centres: facts or fallacies? Am J Orthod 1968;54:566-83.

Laing CJ, Fraser DR. Changes with malnutrition in the concentration of plasma vit. D

binding protein in growing rats. British J Nutr 2002;88:133-9.

Larsen OD, Nielsen A. Mandibular fractures. I. An analysis of their etiology and loca- tion in 286 patients. Scand J Plast Reconstr Surg 1976;10:213-8.

Lê Boff MS, Kohlmeier L, Hurwitz S, Franklin J, Wright J, Glowacki J. Occult vita- min D deficiency in postmenopausal US women with acute hip fracture. JAMA 2000;283:1425-6.

Lindhal L. Condylar fractures of the mandible. I. Classification and relation to age, occlusion; and concomitant injuries of teeth and teeth-supporting structures, and frac- tures of the mandibular body. Int J Oral Surg 1977;6:12-21.

Lindqvist C, Sorsa S, Hyrkas T, Santavirta S. Maxillofacial fractures sustained in bi-cycle accidents. Int J Oral Maxillofac Surg 1986;15:12-8.

Livne E, Silbermann M. The mouse mandibular condyle: an investigative model in developmental biology. J Craniofac Gen Dev Biol 1990;10:95-8.

Luz JGC, Araújo VC. Rotated subcondylar process fracture in the growing animal: an experimental study in rats. Int J Oral Maxillofac Surg 2001;30:545-9.

Luz JGC, Jaeger RG, de Araújo VC, de Rezende JR. The effect of indirect trauma on the rat temporomandibular joint. Int J Oral Maxillofac Surg 1991;20:48-52.

Luz JGC, Rodrigues L. Changes in haemoglobin and haematocrit levels following orthog- nathic surgery of the mandible. Bull Group Int Rech Sci Stomatol Odontol 2004;46:36- 41.

Mabuchi R. The effect of experimental mandibular separation on the mandibular con- dyle in growing rats. Aichi - Gakuin J Dent Sci 1988;26:723-49.

Machado MCC. Malnutrition in the surgical patient. In: Gonçalves EL, Waitzberg DL. Metabolism in surgical practice. São Paulo: Sarvier; 1993.

Manganello-Souza LC, Luz JGC. Fractures of the mandible. In: Manganello-Souza LC, Luz JGC. Surgical treatment of oral and maxillofacial trauma. São Paulo: Roca; 2006. p.189-209.

Markey RJ, Potter BE, Moffett BC. Condylar trauma and facial asymmetry: an experimental study. J

Maxillofac Surg 1980; 8:38-51.

Mellanby RJ, Mellor PJ, Roulois A, Baines EA, Mee AP, Berry JL, et al. Hypocalcae- mia associated with low serum vitamin D metabolite concentrations in two dogs with protein-losing enteropathies. Vet Clin Pathol 2005;34:35-8.

Miller MD, Bannerman E, Daniels LA, Crotty M. Lower limb fracture, cognitive im- pairment and risk of subsequent malnutrition: a prospective evaluation of dietary en- ergy and protein intake on an orthopaedic ward. Eur J Clin Nutr 2006; 60:853-6.

Mitruka BM, Rawnsley HM. Clinical Biochemical and haematological reference values in normal experimental animals. New York: Masson Publishing; 1977.

Miwa T, Shoji H, Solomonow M, Yazdani M, Nakamoto T. The effect of prena- tal protein-energy malnutrition on collagen metabolism in foetal bones. Orthopedics 1989;12:973-7.

Monje F, Delgado E, Navarro MJ, Miralles C, Del Hoyo JRA. Changes in temporoman- dibular joint after mandibular subcondylar osteotomy: an experimental study in rats. J Oral Maxillofac Surg 1993;51:1221-34.

Nakajima V, Kobayasi S, Naresse LE, Leite CVS, Curi PR, Montovani JC. Alterations in the intestinal wall due to protein malnutrition in rats. Evaluation of the rupture strength and the tissue'scollagen. Acta Cir Bras 2008;23:435-40.

Nakamoto T, Miller SA. Physical and biochemical changes of the mandible and long bone in protein-energy malnourished newborn rats. J Nutr 1979a;109:1477-82.

Nakamoto T, Miller SA. The effect of protein-energy malnutrition on the development of bones in newborn rats. J Nutr 1979b; 109:1469-76.

Nakamoto T, Porter JR, Winkler MM. The effect of prenatal protein-energy malnu- trition on the development of mandibles and long bones in newborn rats. Br J Nutr 1983;50:75-80.

Nóbrega FJ. Nutritional disorders. Rio de Janeiro: Revinter; 1998.

Oliveira, LAA. Evaluation of the effect of risedronate sodium on fracture healing. Experimental study in rats. Thesis [Doctorate]. São Paulo: USP Medical School; 2003.

Oliveira TRC, Frigerio MLMA. Nutritional and protein evaluation of edentulous senes- cents - a comparative study between patients with mucosal-supported-implant-retained total prostheses and conventional total prostheses. RPG 2005; 12:255-63.

Ortega-Flores CI, Costa MALC, Cereda MP, Penteado MDVC. Evaluation of the protein quality of dehydrated cassava leaf (Manohot esculenta Crantz). Nutrire Rev Soc Bras Aliment Nutr 2003;25:47-59.

Pallaro AN, Roux ME, Slobodianik NH. Nutrition disorders and immunologic parameters: study of the thymus in growing rats. Nutr 2001;17:724-8.

Pellet PL, Young VR. Nutritional evaluation of protein foods. Tokyo: The United Nations University; 1980. 62 p.

Pinkert R. Histologische Untersuchungen uber das verhalten des Discus bei Frakturen des Processus condylaris des Unterkiefers. Stomat DDR 1982;32:27-32.

Pompeo M. Misconceptions about protein requeriments for wound healing: results of a prospective study. Ostomy/Wound Management 2007;53:30-44.

Porto G, Vasconcelos B, Silva Junior V. Development of temporomandibular joint anky- losis in rats: a preliminary experimental study. J Oral Maxillofac Surg 2008; 37:282-6.

Prentice A, Schoenmakers I, Laskey MA, de Bono S, Ginty F, Goldberg GR. Nutrition and bone growth and development. Proc Nutr Soc 2006;65:348-60.

Prestes-Carneiro LE, Laraya RD, Silva PRC, Moliterno RA, Felipe I, Mathias PC. Long-term effect of early protein malnutrition on growth curve, haematological pa- rameters and macrophage function of rats. J Nutr Sci Vitaminol 2006;52:414-20.

Proffit WR, Vig KWL, Turvey TA. Early fracture of the mandibular condyles: frequently an unsuspected cause of growth disturbances. Amer J Orthod 1980; 78:1-24.

Ribeiro Passos de Oliveira S, Martins Bion F, Limongi Lopes SM, Cavalcanti Metri A. Use of food mixture containing bioproteins (saccharomyces cerevisiae): effects on gestation, lactation and growth of rats. Arch. latinoam Nutr 2001;51:72- 80.

Rocha FMVF, Goulart AC, Novelli MD, Luz JGC. Effects of zygomatic arch fracture on facial growth in young rats. Rev Odontol Univ São Paulo 1999;13: 37-41.

Rodrigues L, Luz JGC. Consequences of mandibular condyle removal on maxillary and mandibular growth: experimental study in rats. Acta Cir Bras 2001 Jan-Mar; 16(1). Available from: URL: http:/www.scielo.br/acb.

Rodrigues L, Luz, JGC, Miori CA. Analysis of the haemogram and blood biochemistry of patients with facial fractures. RPG Fac Odontol Univ São Paulo 1999;6:278. res. 5.

Rodrigues RL, Zucas SM. Influence of energy-protein malnutrition on bone callus formation: a radiological study. Rev Bras Ortop 1991;26:67-73.

Sanderson JH, Philips CE. An atlas of laboratory animal haematology. New York: Oxford University Press; 1981.

SanflAna DMG, Molinari SL, Miranda Neto MH. Effects of protein and vitamin B defi- ciency on blood parameters and myemteric neurons of the colon of rats. Arq Neurop- sychiatr 2001;59:493-98.

Santos MAS, Ferraz MR, Teixeira CV, Sampaio FJB, Fontes Ramos C. Effects of under- nutrition on serum and testicular testosterone levels and sexual function in adult rats. Horm Metab Res 2004;36:27-33.

Seebeck P, Bail HJ, Exner C, Schell H, Michel R, Amthauer H, et al. Do serological tissue turnover markers represent callus formation during fracture healing? Bone 2005;37:669-77.

Sgarbieri VC. Proteins in protein foods: properties - degradations - modifications. São Paulo: Varela; 1996. p.337-42.

Sheiham A, Steele JG, Marcenes W, Lowe C, Finch S, Bates CJ. et al. The relationship among dental status, nutrient intake, and nutritional status in older people. J Dent Res 2001;80:408-13.

Shimahara M, Ono K, Nakano Y. An experimental study on intermaxillary fixation in the healing process of fracture of the condylar process of the mandible. Bull Osaka Med Sch 1985;31:42-55.

Shimahara M, Ono K, Terai A, Konda T, Toyoshima A, Yonenaga T. An experimental study on the healing of fracture of the condylar process of the mandible - the course after malunion. Bull Osaka Med Sch 1987;33:164-78.

Silvennoinen V, Iizukat T, Lindquist C, Oikarinen K. Different patterns of condy- lar fractures: an analysis of 382 patients in a 3 - year period. J Oral Maxillofac Surg 1992;50:1032-37.

Sprinz R. Healing of fractures of the neck of the mandible in rats with detachment of the lateral pterygoid muscle. Arch Oral Biol 1970;15:1219-29.

Stark AD, Bennet GC, Stone DH. Association between childhood fractures and poverty: population based study. BMJ 2002;23:324-457.

Suuronen R, Vainionpaa S, Hietanen J, Vasenius J, Lindquist C. The effect of osteoto- my and osteosynthesis in the mandibular condyle. A radiological and histological study in sheep. Int J Oral Maxillofac Surg 1994;23:174-79.

Takatsuka S, Terai K, Yoshida K, Narinobou M, Ueki K, Nakagawa K, et al. A com- parative study of unilateral dislocated mandibular condyle fractures in the rabbit. J Cranio-Maxillofac Surg 2005;33:180-187.

Teixeira AC, Luz JG, Araújo VC, Araújo NS. Healing of the displaced condylar process fracture: an experimental study. J Cranio Maxillofac Surg 1998;26:326-30.

Teixeira VCB, Teixeira ACB, Luz JGC. Skeletal changes after experimentally displaced condylar process fracture in growing rats. J Cranio-Maxillofac Surg 2006;34:220-25.

Thaller SR, Reavie D, Daniller A. Rigid internal fixation with miniplates and screws: a cost-effective technique for treating mandible fractures? Ann Plast Surg 1990;24:469- 74.

UNICEF. World situation of children. Brasilia: UNICEF; 1994.

Vannucchi H, Unamuno M do R Dell de, Marchini JS. Assessment of nutritional status. Medicina Ribeirão Preto. 1996; 29:5-18.

Who. Expert committee on nutrition. 6th report.1962. (Who technical report series, 45).

Winstanley RP. The management of fractures of the mandible. Br J Oral Maxillofac Surg 1984;22:170-77.

Yamamoto MK, Novelli MD, Luz JGC. Effects of unilateral upper incisor extraction on facial growth of young rats. J Nihon Univ Sch Dent 1997,39:191-5.

Yasuoka T, Oka N. Histomorphometric study of trabecular bone remodelling during condylar process fracture healing in the growing period: experimental study. J Oral Maxillofac Surg 1991;49:981-8.

Yunes J. Predisposing factors, incidence and prevalence, mortality and morbidity. In: Marcondes E. Desnutrição. São Paulo: Sarvier; 1976. p. 31.

Zanin STM. Morphological and quantitative study of the myenteric plexus of the duodenum of rats submitted to a hypoprotein diet and deficient in B vitamins. [Master's dissertation]. São Paulo: USP Biomedical Sciences Institute; 2003.

Zheng L, Yamashiro T, Fukunaga T, Balam TA, Takano-Yamamoto T. Bone morpho- genetic protein 3 expression pattern in rat condylar cartilage, femoral cartilage and mandibular fracture callus. Eur J Oral Sei 2005;113:318-25.

ANNEX A - Research Ethics Committee opinion

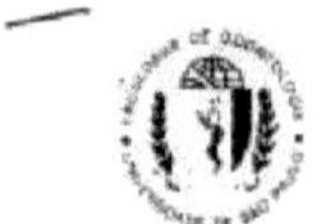

UNIVERSIDADE DE SÃO PAULO
FACULDADE DE ODONTOLOGIA

PARECER DE APROVAÇÃO
PROTOCOLO nº 08/05

Com base em parecer de relator, o Comitê de Ética em Pesquisa – Subcomissão de Bioética de Animais da FOUSP, **APROVOU** o protocolo de pesquisa ***"Avaliação das alterações anatomofuncionais locais e sistêmicas em ratos (Rattus norvegicus) submetidos a fratura condilar: estudo da influência de fatores nutricionais no processo de reparação óssea"***, de responsabilidade da pesquisadora **Luciana Corrêa**, sob orientação do Professor Doutor **João Gualberto de Cerqueira Luz.**

Cabe ao responsável enviar relatórios referentes ao andamento da pesquisa após 06 (seis) meses e 01(um) ano desta data, bem como cópia do trabalho em "cd" ou "disquete" ao finalizá-lo, conforme legislação vigente.

São Paulo, 14 de junho de 2005

Prof. Dr. Celso Luiz Caldeira
Presidente da Subcomissão de Bioética de Animais da FOUSP

ANNEX B

Table 1- Composition of normal and low-protein diets

Nutrient	Diet	
	Normoprotein	Hypoprotein
Total energy - kcal	4070.4	4070.4
Protein %	23.0	8.0
Carbohydrates %	66.0	81.0
Lipids %	11.0	11.0
Protein g	230.0	80.0
Carbohydrates g	676.0	826.0
Lipids g	50.0	50.0
Vitamin Mix g	4.0	4.0
Mixture of Mineral Salts g	40.0	40.0

*According to the recommendations of the American Institute of Nutrition Rodents Diets, AIN-93G (1993).

ANNEX C

Table 2 - Composition of the vitamin mixture

Vitamins*	g/kg of mixture
Nicotinic Acid	3.000
Pantothenic Acid	1.600
Pyridoxine - B6	0.700
Thiamine - B1	0.600
Riboflavin	0.600
Folic Acid	0.200
Biotin	0.020
Cyanocobalamin - B12	2.500
Vitamin E (500 IU/g)	15.00
Vitamin A (500,000 IU/g)	0.800
Vitamin D (400,000 IU/g)	0.250
Vitamin K	0.075

*According to the recommendations of the American Institute of Nutrition Rodents Diets, AIN-93G (1993).

ANNEX D

Table 3 - Composition of the mineral mixture

Minerals *	g/kg of mixture
Calcium carbonate, 40.04% Ca	357.00
Potassium Phosphate, 22.76% P; 28.73% K	196.00
Potassium Citrate, 36.16% K	70.78
Sodium Chloride, 39.34% Na; 60.66% Cl	74.00
Potassium sulphate, 44.87% K; 18.39% S	46.60
Magnesium oxide, 60.32% Mg	24.00
Iron Citrate, 16.5% Fe	6.06
Zinc carbonate, 52.14% Zn	1.65
Manganese carbonate, 47.79% Mn	0.63
Copper carbonate, 57.47% Cu	0.30
Potassium Iodide, 59.3% I	0.01
Sodium Selenate, 41.79% Se	0.010
Ammonium Paramolybidate, 54.34% Mo	0.008

*According to the recommendations of the American Institute of Nutrition Rodents Diets, AIN-

93G (1993).

ANNEX E

Table 4 - Vitamins used to make the hypoprotein feed

Vitamin	Quantity
B complex	1ml
B12	10 pl
vitamin K	75 pl
Aderogil® (vitamins A and D)	1 ml
vitamin E	1 drop

ANNEX F

Groups	24 hours	7 days	15 days	30 days	90 days
Fractured group	1 day	1 week	2 weeks	4 weeks	12 weeks
Fractured and malnourished group	4 weeks + 1 day	4 weeks + 1 week	4 weeks + 2 weeks	4 weeks + 4 weeks	4 weeks + 12 weeks
Malnourished group	4 weeks + 1 day	4 weeks + 1 week	4 weeks + 2 weeks	4 weeks + 4 weeks	4 weeks + 12 weeks

Table 1 - Total weeks used as a basis for calculating feed consumption and EAA.

ANNEX G

Table 7 - Average weight values (g) of the animals in the different groups and experimental periods

Period	Fractured group (F)			Fractured group malnourished (FD)			Malnourished group (D)		
	In	Fr	Sacr.	In	Fr	Sacr	In	Fr	Sacr
24 hours	336	336	321	273,9	296,3	306,3	296,7	*	338,9
7 days	286,3	286,3	312,3	336,5	380,8	332,5	276,5	*	309,3
15 days	283,1	283,1	302,1	354,3	374,5	335,5	312	*	372,9
30 days	279	279	308,4	309,7	367,9	363,9	297	*	372,5
90 days	307,6	307,6	432,3	315	347	365,5	257,3	*	400,5

In - start of experiment (time zero); Fr - day of fracture; Sacr - day of sacrifice

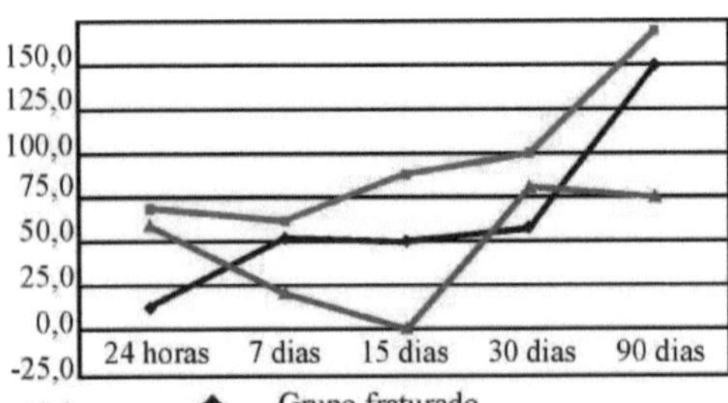

Graph 1 - Average rate of weight gain or loss according to experimental periods

ANNEX H

Table 5 - Values of the biochemical tests carried out on the animals in the negative control group (without fracture and without malnutrition) and reference values from Mitruka and Rawnsley (1977)

	Total protein (g/dL)	Albumin (g/dL)	Calcium (mg/dL)	Alkaline phosphatase (U/L)	Serum iron g/(udL)	Creatinine k(mg/dL)
Negative control	5,55±0,44	1,98±0,04	9,93±0,11	45,98±14,21	222,46±24,31	0,61±0,42
Reference values	4.7-8.15	2.7-5.1	7.2-13.9	56.8-128	-	0.2-0.8

ANNEX I

Table 6 - Normal leucogram data for adult male rats

Age of the animals	CGL (x103/mm3)	Neutrophils (x109/l)	Eosinophils (x109/l)	Monocytes (x109/l)	Lymphocytes (x109/l)	Basophils (x109/l)
26 weeks	3,7 a 8,7	0,3 a 2,4	0,0 a 0,2	0,0 a 0,7	3,0 a 6,4	0,0 a 0,0
52 weeks	3,3 a 8,3	0,5 a 3,4	0,0 a 0,1	0,0 a 0,2	1,9 a 6,7	0,0 a 0,0

Adapted from Sanderson and Philips (1981). SANDERSON, J.H.; PHILIPS, C.E. An atlas of laboratory animal haematology. NewYork : Oxford University Press, 1981

ANNEX J

Table 2 - Average total leucocyte count values (x103/mm3) by group and period

period	F (x103/mm3)	FD (x103/mm3)	D (x103/mm3)
24 hours	5.07±2.02	8.63±2.1	4.2±2.36
7 days	3.23±0.6	12.73±2.72	4.47±1.34
15 days	4.13±0.85	5.57±1.15	3.80±0.7
30 days	6.37±4.6	11.53±4.11	4.27±2.05
90 days	3.97±0.67	6.17±2.49	4.00±1.99

Reference values- Negative control :3.6±1.5 x103/mm3 ;
SANDERSON; PHILIPS, 1981 : 3.3 to 8.3 x103/mm3

Table 3 - Mean values (%) of individual leucocyte counts in the groups per period

Cells	24 hours (%)			7 days (%)			15 days (%)		
	F	FD	D	F	FD	D	F	FD	D
Lymphocytes	73.0 ± 1.0	66.67a ±4.0	85.3b ±1.5	71.3 ±3.5	65.3a ±8.6	84.3b ±4.1	58.7 ±13.0	66.7 ±12.0	76.0 ±2.6
Monocytes	2.7 ±1.1	1.7 ±2.0	1.0 ±0.0	2.7 ±2.5	1.3 ±1.1	1.3 ±1.1	1.3 ±1.5	0.3 ±0.6	2.7 ±1.9
Neutrophils	23.3 ±1.5	30.7a ±5.0	13.7b ±1.5	26.0 ±3.6	33.3a ±8.5	13.3b ±3.0	36.7 ±17.6	33.0 ±11.5	20.3 ±3.2
Eosinophils	0	0	0	0	0	1	0	0	0
Basophils	0	0	0	0	0	0	0	0	0
Rods	0	1	0	0	0	0	0	0	0
	30 days (%)			**90 days (%)**			**Reference Values**		

Cells	F	FD	D	F	FD	D	Negative control	Mitruka & Rawnsley (1977)
Lymphocytes	79.3[a] ±0.6	76.0 ±5.6	70.3b ±1.5	79.0 ±1.0	82.0 ±9.2	75.7 ±3.2	72,0±4.6	57,0-83,0
Monocytes	0.7 ±0.6	2.7 ±3.8	1.3 ±0.9	1.0 ±0.0	1.0 ±1.0	1.7 ±0.5	1.3±0.6	0,0-0,65
Neutrophils	20.0 ±1.0	21.3 ±7.6	25.3 ±5.0	18.0 ±1.0	17.0 ±10.1	19.7 ±2.5	26.0±5.3	6.0-42.0
Eosinophils	0	0	0	0	0	0	0,3±0,6	0,09-0,63
Basophils	0	0	0	0	0	0	0,0±0,0	
Rods	0	0	0	0	0	0	0,0±0,0	

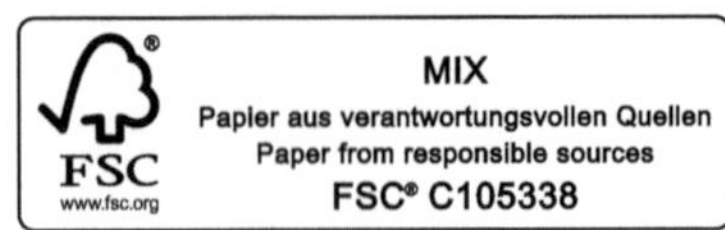

Printed by Books on Demand GmbH, Norderstedt / Germany